Tasty Therapeutic Recipes

Wholesome Meals for Healing, Rejuvenation, and Fun

BY: Martin Beasant

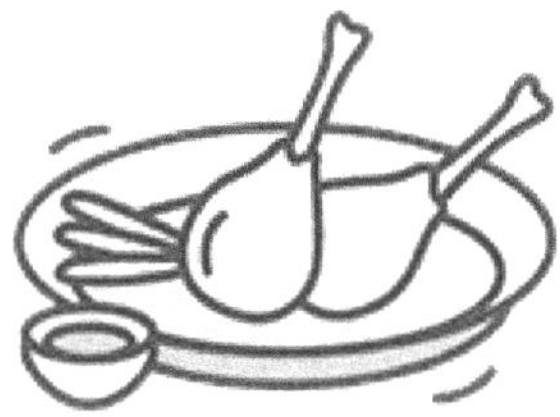

Notification Page

Hello there,

I kindly request that you refrain from reproducing this book in any form, whether it be printed or electronic, sold, published, disseminated or distributed without obtaining prior written permission from the author.

I have taken great care in ensuring that the content of this book is accurate and helpful, but it is the reader's responsibility to exercise caution in their actions. Please note that the author cannot be held responsible for any consequences resulting from the reader's actions.

Thank you for your understanding and cooperation.

Sincerely,

Martin Beasant

Table of Contents

Introduction

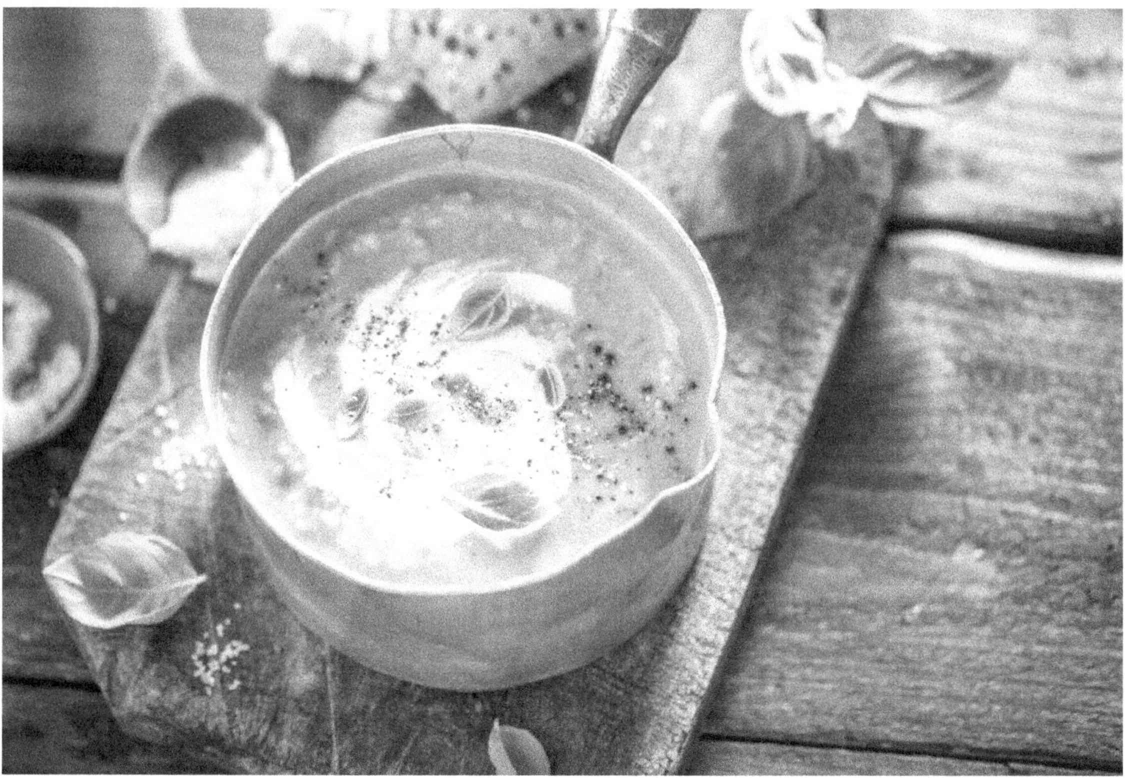

For a moment of healing, de-stressing, and unwinding, cooking is a proven activity to practice. Engaging in the art of creating delicious meals, playing with colorful ingredients, and embracing the individual steps of bringing a full meal to life is a beautiful stride towards feeling refreshed and whole.

Adding to that would be choosing meals that aren't only a delight to cook but pack essential nutrients that help your body heal. Lots of greens, vegetables, fruits, seeds, protein, and healthy fats are perfect choices to consider.

While at that, to ensure that the flavor and taste turnouts are fantastic, we assembled these thirty recipes that are perfect for therapy cooking. From breakfast to dessert, these meals are a delight to make and would make you feel better than you started.

1. High Protein Savory Breakfast Muffins

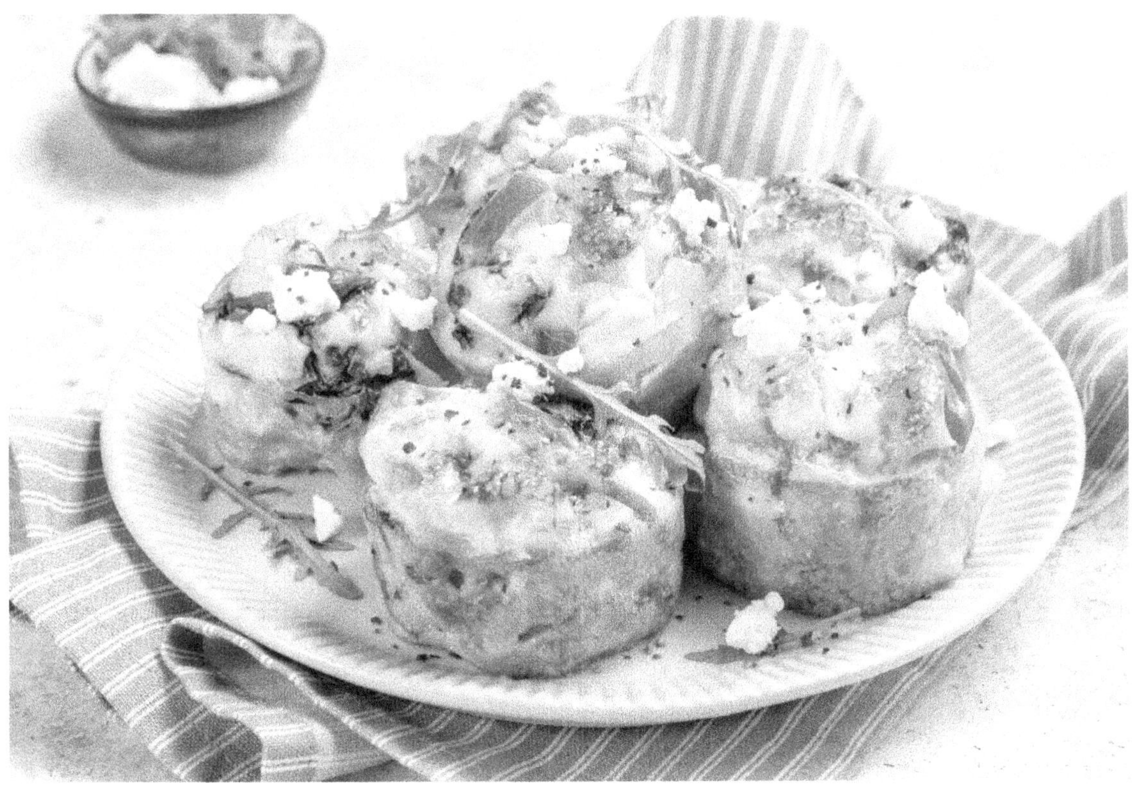

Enriched with turkey, cottage cheese, and eggs, these savory muffins are awesome for a good morning start.

Prep Time: 20 mins

Cook Time: 25 mins

Serves: 12

Ingredients:

- 1 cup 2% cottage cheese
- 4 eggs
- 1 lb. turkey breakfast sausages, removed from the casing
- ¼ cup milk
- 1 tbsp olive oil
- Kosher salt and black pepper to taste
- 1 ½ cups almond flour
- 2 tsp baking powder
- 3 cups chopped mixed vegetables (bell peppers, broccoli, spinach etc.)
- 3 green onions greens and whites, thinly sliced
- 1 cup shredded cheddar cheese

Instructions:

1. Preheat the oven to 400°F. Grease a 12-cup muffin tin.
2. Brown the turkey in a skillet over medium heat for 5 minutes. Transfer to a plate.
3. Beat the eggs with the milk, olive oil, cottage cheese, salt, and black pepper. Whisk in the flour and baking powder until smooth. Mix in the vegetables, green onions, and cheddar cheese.
4. Fill the muffin tin holes three-fourth way up. Bake for 20 to 25 minutes or until baked through. Serve the egg muffins warm.

2. Homemade Cocoa Granola

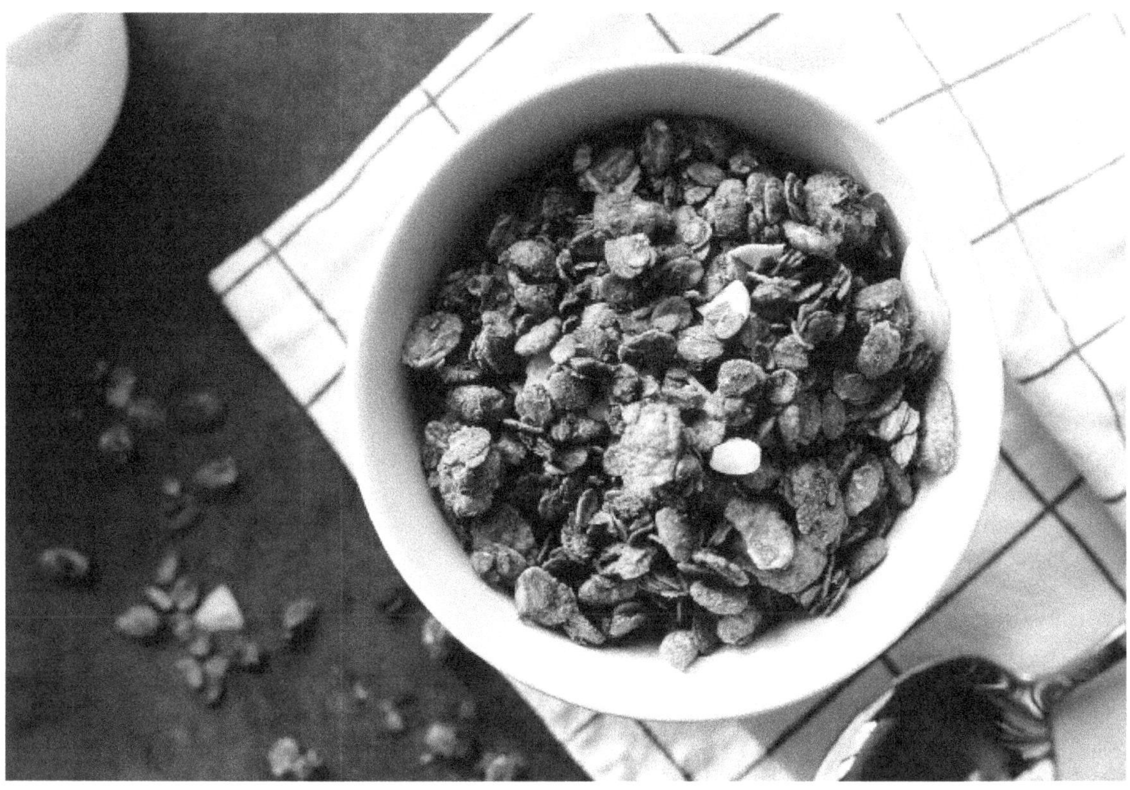

Enjoy a guilt-free treat that is chocolate-enriched granola for a pleasurable breakfast that is nutrient-packed too.

Prep Time: 10 mins

Cook Time: 24 mins

Serves: 9 (½ cup servings)

Ingredients:

- 3 cups gluten-free rolled oats
- ¼ cup unsweetened shredded coconut
- 1 cup chopped raw nuts (almonds, walnuts, pecans), roughly chopped
- ⅓ cup cocoa powder
- 2 tbsp chia seeds
- 3 tbsp coconut or organic cane sugar
- 1 tsp sea salt
- ¼ cup coconut oil or other healthy oil of choice
- ½ cup maple syrup or honey
- ½ cup sweet dark chocolate chips or chunks

Instructions:

1. Preheat the oven to 340°F. Line a baking sheet with baking paper.
2. Mix the oats, coconut, nuts, cocoa powder, chia seeds, sugar, and salt in a bowl. Heat the oil and maple syrup or honey in a small saucepan over low heat; pour over the oats mixture. Mix well.
3. Spread the mixture on the baking sheet and bake for 17 to 24 minutes or until golden brown and fragrant.
4. Let the granola cool completely. Stir in the chocolate once cooled. Preserve in an airtight container at room temperature.

3. Strawberry Banana Bread

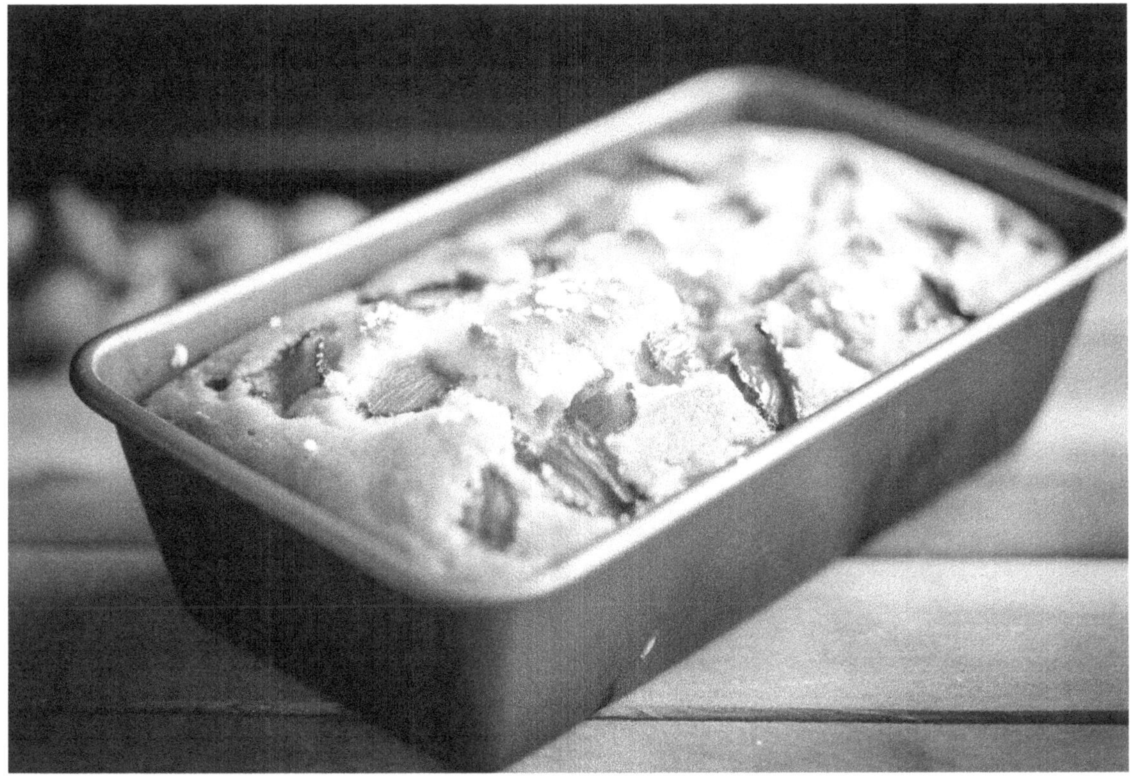

Strawberries add a beautiful color to cinnamon-banana bread for sweet, soft bites.

Prep Time: 20 mins

Cook Time: 80 mins

Serves: 12

Ingredients:

- 2 ½ cups all-purpose flour
- 1 tsp ground cinnamon
- ½ tsp salt
- 1 tsp baking soda
- ½ cup unsalted butter, softened
- ¾ cup granulated sugar
- ¾ cup sour cream
- 2 large eggs, at room temperature
- 1 tsp vanilla extract
- 3 medium ripe bananas, mashed
- 2 cups strawberries, thinly sliced, divided
- 1 cup chopped nuts of choice

Instructions:

1. Preheat the oven to 350°F. Grease a 9 x 5-inch loaf pan with cooking spray and line it with baking paper. Set aside.
2. Mix the flour, baking soda, cinnamon, and salt in a bowl. Cream the butter and sugar in another bowl. Whisk in the sour cream, eggs, and vanilla. Gradually mix in the flour mixture until smooth. Mix in the mashed bananas and fold in 1 ½ cups of strawberries and nuts. Pour the batter into the loaf pan and arrange the remaining strawberries in the batter.
3. Bake for 60 to 80 minutes or until golden brown and baked through at the center. Cool in the pan for 10 minutes. Transfer the bread to a wire rack to cool completely. Slice and serve.

4. High Fiber Seed Bread

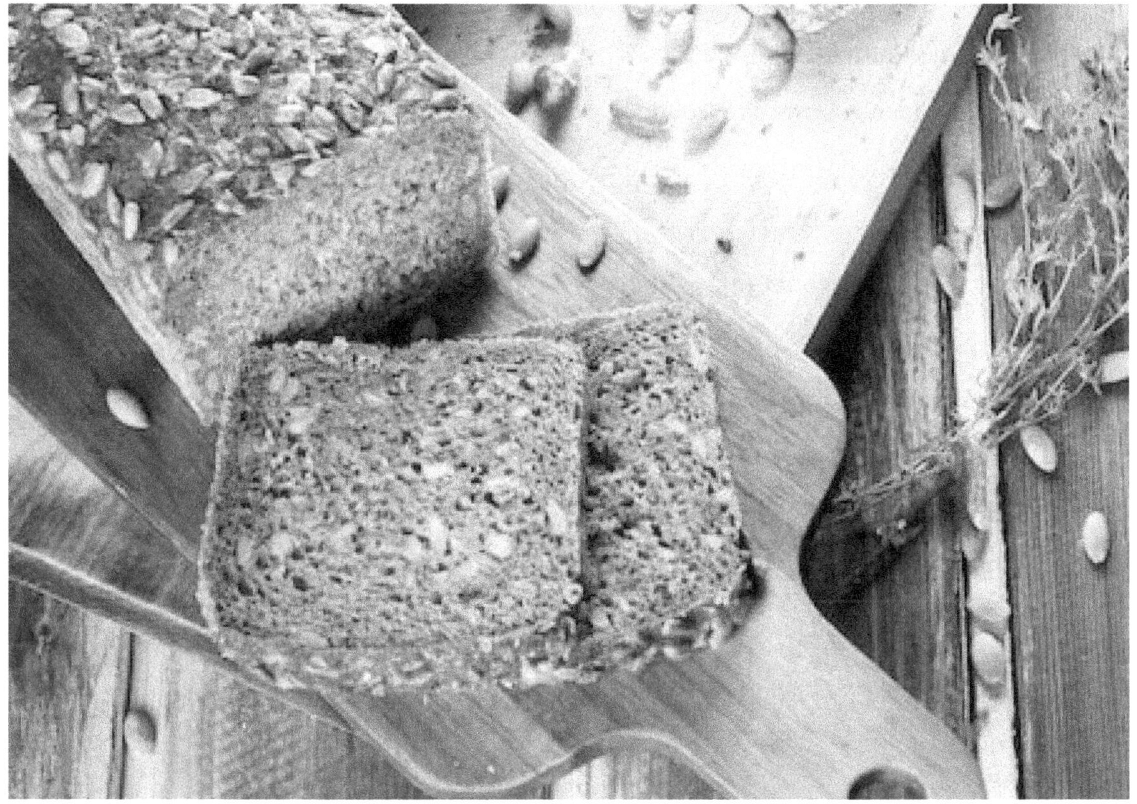

Great for the tummy and super packed with nutrients, you'll feel refreshed and restored after a slice.

Prep Time: 20 mins

Cook Time: 45 mins

Serves: 12

Ingredients:

- 1 ½ cups oat flour
- 4 tbsp psyllium husk powder
- ½ cup golden flax seeds, ground
- 2 tbsp chia seeds, ground
- 1 tsp sea salt
- 3 tbsp refined coconut oil, melted
- ⅓ cup date syrup
- ½ cups warm water about 100°F, divided
- ¼ cup dried cherries or raisins for less tartness, soaked with the dates
- ½ cup almonds, coarsely chopped
- ½ cup hazelnuts or macadamia nuts, coarsely chopped
- ½ cup pumpkin seeds
- 1 cup sunflower seeds

Instructions:

1. Preheat the oven to 350°F. Grease a 9 x 5-inch loaf pan with cooking spray and line it with baking paper. Set aside.
2. Mix the oat flour, psyllium husk powder, flax seeds, chia seeds, and salt in a bowl. Mix in the coconut oil, date syrup, and warm water until smooth batter forms. Fold in cherries or raisins, nuts, and seeds. Pour the batter into the loaf pan.
3. Bake for 45 minutes or until baked through. Cool in the pan for 10 minutes. Transfer the bread to a wire rack to cool completely. Slice and serve.

5. Matcha Green Smoothie

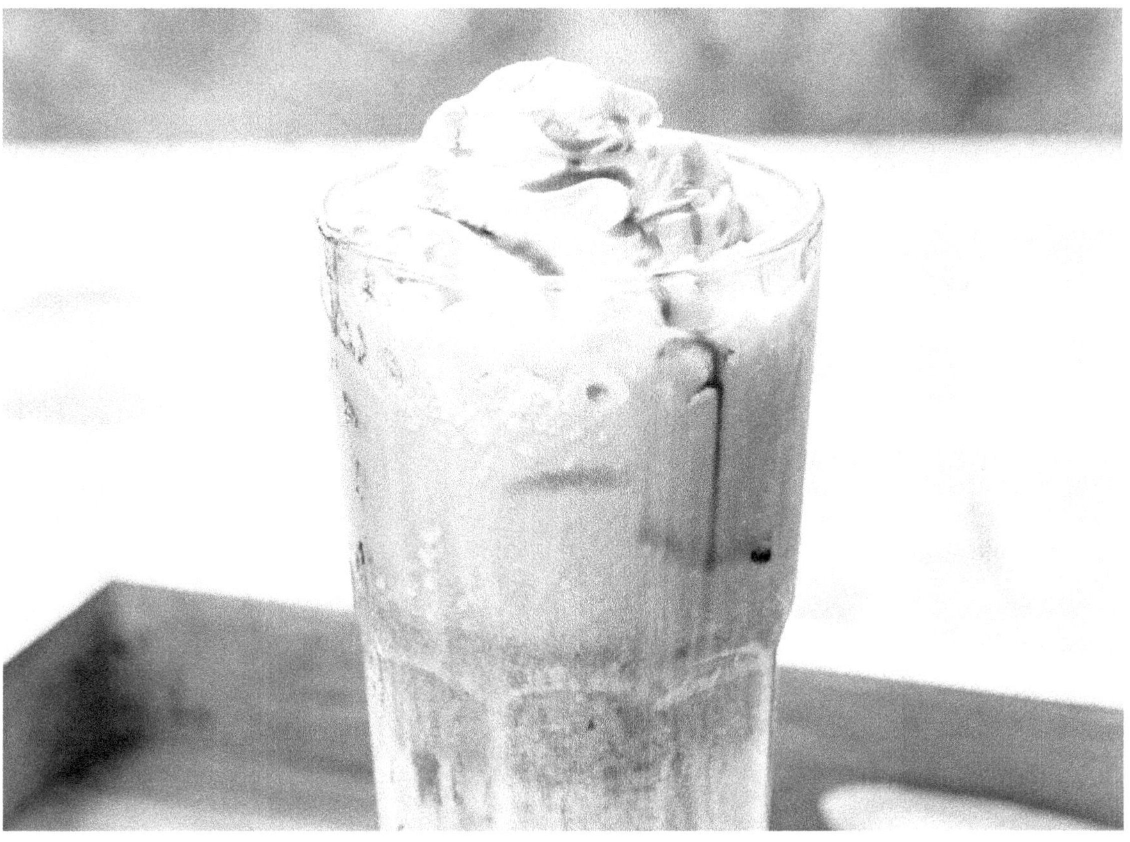

Thoroughly healthy and smooth on the swallow, matcha green tea powder and raw greens combine in this yummy smoothie.

Prep Time: 10 mins

Serves: 4

Ingredients:

- 2 cups ice cubes
- ½ cup nonfat plain Greek yogurt, or dairy-free
- 1 cup unsweetened almond milk
- 1 banana, peeled and sliced
- 1 cup baby spinach
- 1 cup baby kale
- ¼ cup sliced almonds
- 1 tbsp matcha green tea powder
- 2 tsp honey or maple syrup

Instructions:

1. Add all the ingredients to a blender. Blend until smooth.
2. Pour into glasses and enjoy!

6. Baobab Green Juice

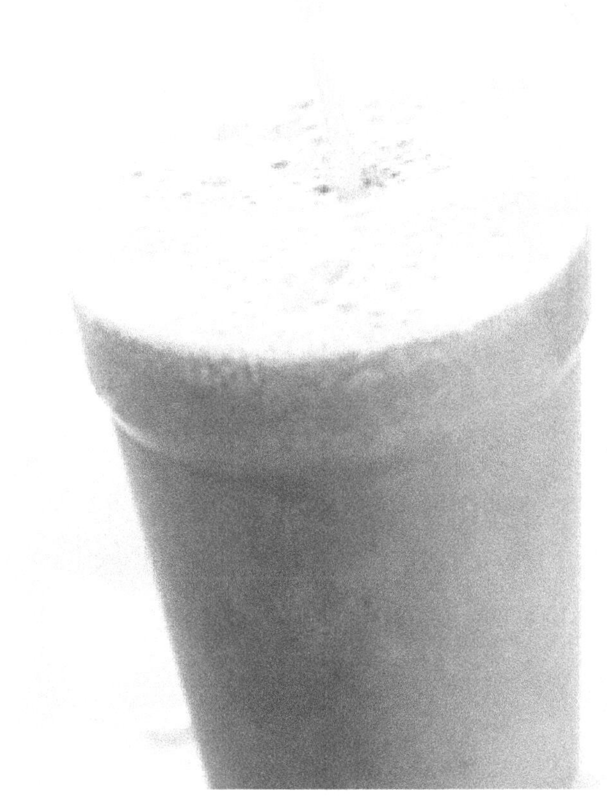

A calming juice packed with vitamin C to boost the immune system. Enjoy it as a summer refresher over ice.

Prep Time: 10 mins

Serves: 4 (1 cup servings)

Ingredients:

- 1 lemongrass stalk, trimmed, pale green parts only
- 2 green apples, halved
- 2 tsp baobab powder
- 1 small green cabbage, outer leaves removed, cut into small wedges
- 1 medium fennel bulb, cored and quartered
- 4 celery stalks
- 1 (2-inch) piece ginger, peeled

Instructions:

1. Using a juicer, juice the cabbage, lemongrass, apples, fennel, celery, and ginger. Pour the juice into an airtight container and refrigerate until cold.
2. When ready to serve, stir in the baobab powder. Serve the drink over ice in glasses.

7. Blueberry-Banana Smoothie with Tahini

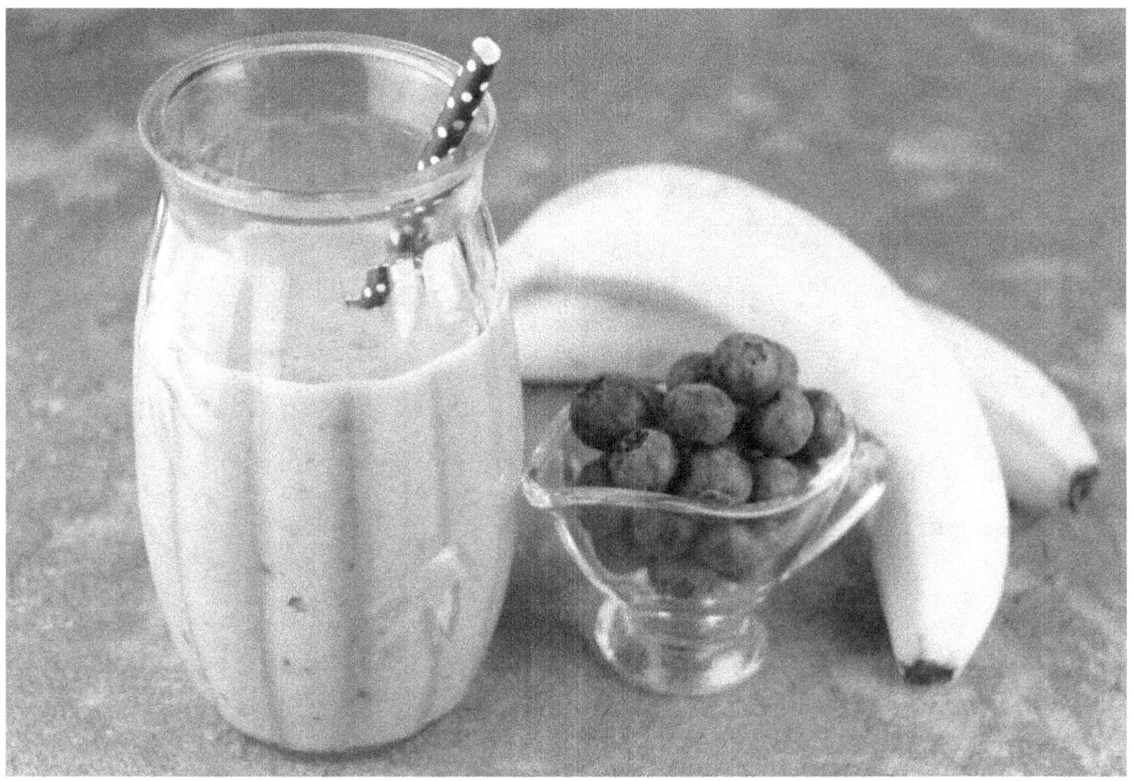

Each sip is rewarding and restoring. Bananas, blueberries, and sesame taste so good together.

Prep Time: 10 mins

Cook Time: 8 mins

Serves: 4

Ingredients:

- 1 cup frozen blueberries
- 1 fresh banana, peeled, cut into large pieces,
- ¼ cup tahini
- 1 cup nut milk
- A pinch of ground cinnamon
- ½ tsp vanilla extract

Instructions:

1. Add all the ingredients to a blender. Blend until smooth.
2. Pour into glasses and enjoy!

8. Curried Tomato, Lentil, and Coconut Soup

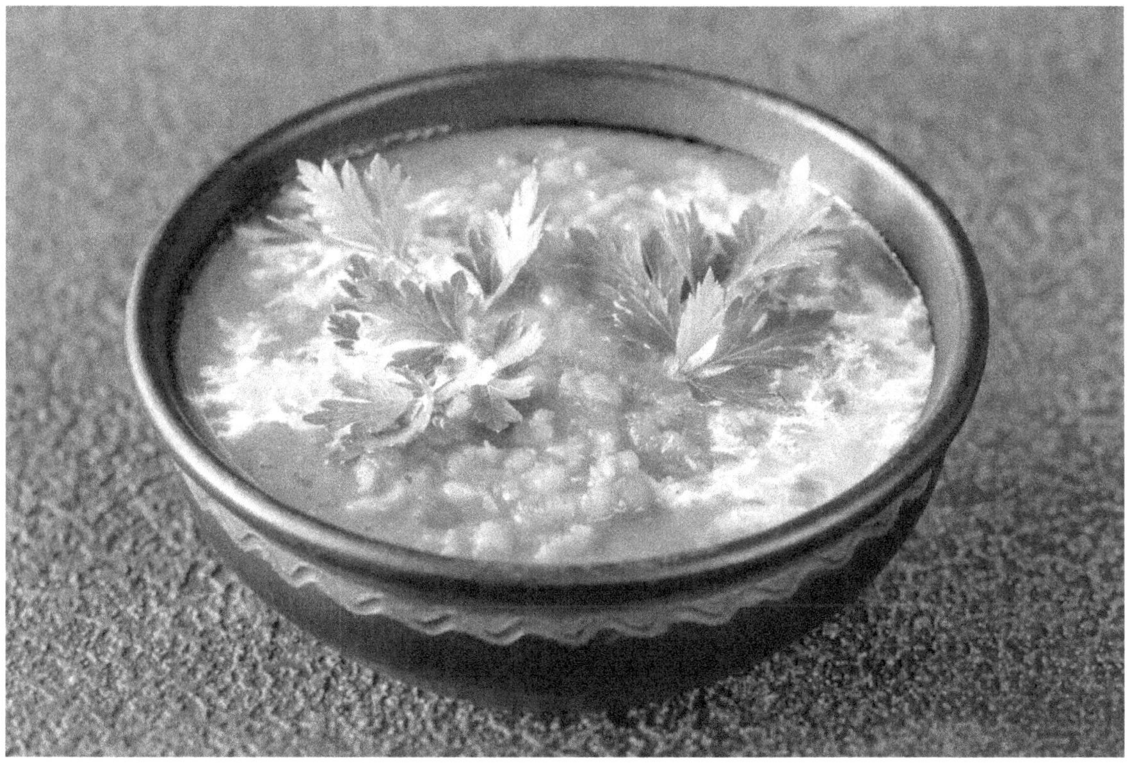

Cuddle up with a hearty bowl of softened lentils cooked in tomatoes and coconut milk. An excellent warmer for the cold days.

Prep Time: 10 mins

Freeze Time: 30 mins

Serves: 4

Ingredients:

- 2 tbsp extra-virgin olive oil or coconut oil
- 1 medium onion, finely chopped
- 2 garlic cloves, minced
- 1 (2 ½-inch) piece ginger, peeled and finely grated
- ¼ tsp crushed red pepper flakes
- 1 tbsp medium curry powder
- ¾ cup red lentils
- 1 (14.5 oz) can crushed tomatoes
- ½ cup finely chopped fresh cilantro, plus extra for serving
- Lime wedges for serving
- Kosher salt and black pepper to taste
- 1 (13.5 oz) can unsweetened coconut milk, shaken well

Instructions:

1. Heat the oil in a large saucepan over medium heat. Sauté the onion for 3 minutes or until tender. Sauté the garlic, ginger, red pepper flakes, and curry powder for 1 minute or until fragrant. Stir in the red lentils and cook for 1 minute. Stir in the cilantro, tomatoes, salt, black pepper, and all but ¼ cup of the coconut milk. Bring to a boil and then simmer over low heat for 20 to 25 minutes or until the lentils are soft. Adjust the taste with salt and black pepper.
2. Dish the soup in bowls topped with the reserved coconut milk and garnished with cilantro. Serve with lime wedges.

9. Chicken and Spelt Soup with Greens

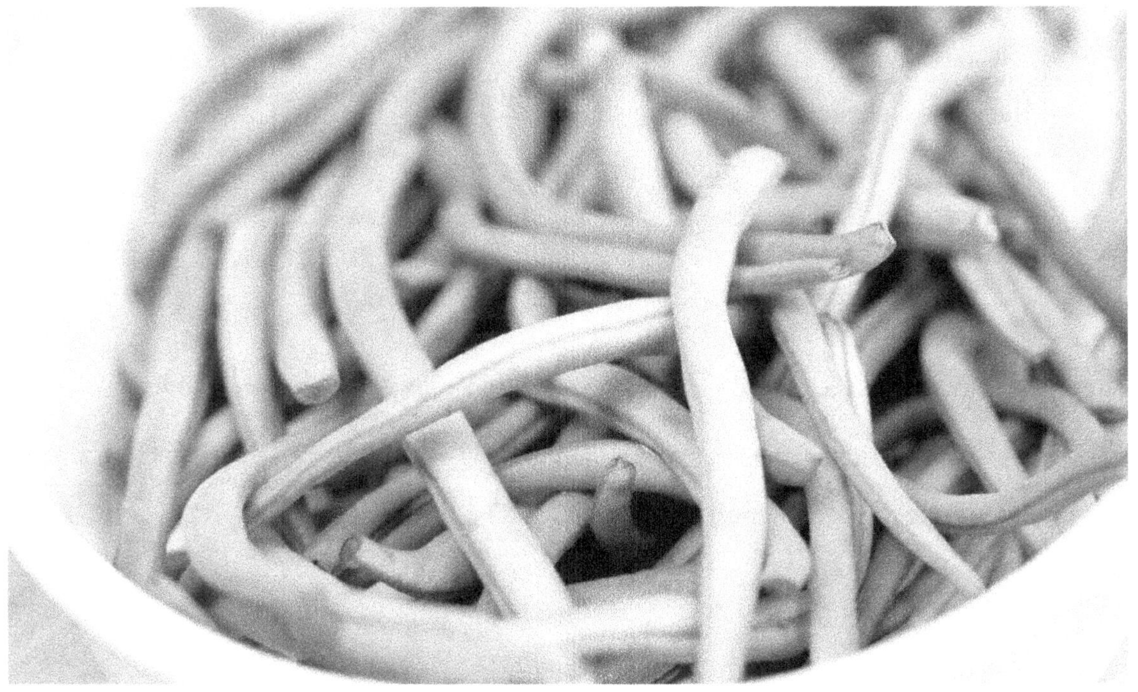

This soup works great for reusing leftover chicken and giving it a healthy bang. Cooked with spelt, greens, and even more veggies, it is an instant energy boost.

Prep Time: 20 mins

Cook Time: 1 hour 56 mins

Serves: 4

Ingredients:

- 1 carrot, peeled and chopped
- 1 leek, chopped
- Baby lemon balm leaves to garnish
- 3.5 oz green beans, trimmed and chopped
- 1 tsp black peppercorns
- ¾ cup baby kale leaves
- 2 liters water
- 3 stalks celery, chopped, divided
- 1 (3 ¼ lb.) chicken, rinsed and drained
- 1 tbsp finely grated lemon zest
- 1 cup spelt
- 1 yellow onion, skin on, quartered
- 2 fresh bay leaves
- Kosher salt and cracked black pepper to taste
- 10.5 oz broccolini, florets trimmed and stalk chopped
- 1 head garlic, halved crosswise

Instructions:

1. Add the chicken, carrot, onion, 1 celery, leek, garlic, bay leaves, black peppercorns, and water to a large pot. Bring to boil over high heat and then simmer covered over low heat for 1 hour 30 minutes. Next, strain the soup, reserving the stock and chicken. Discard the other elements.

2. Return the stock to the pot, add the spelt, and boil over high heat. Reduce the heat to medium and cook covered for 15 minutes or until the spelt is tender. Meanwhile, shred the chicken, set it aside, and discard the bones or use them for chicken stock.

3. Add the remaining celery, broccolini, salt, and black pepper; cook for 4 minutes. Stir in the green beans and chicken; cook for 2 minutes or until the green beans are tender. Turn the heat off and stir in the kale and lemon zest.

4. Dish the soup garnished with lemon balm and cracked black pepper.

10. Spicy Fisherman Fish Stew

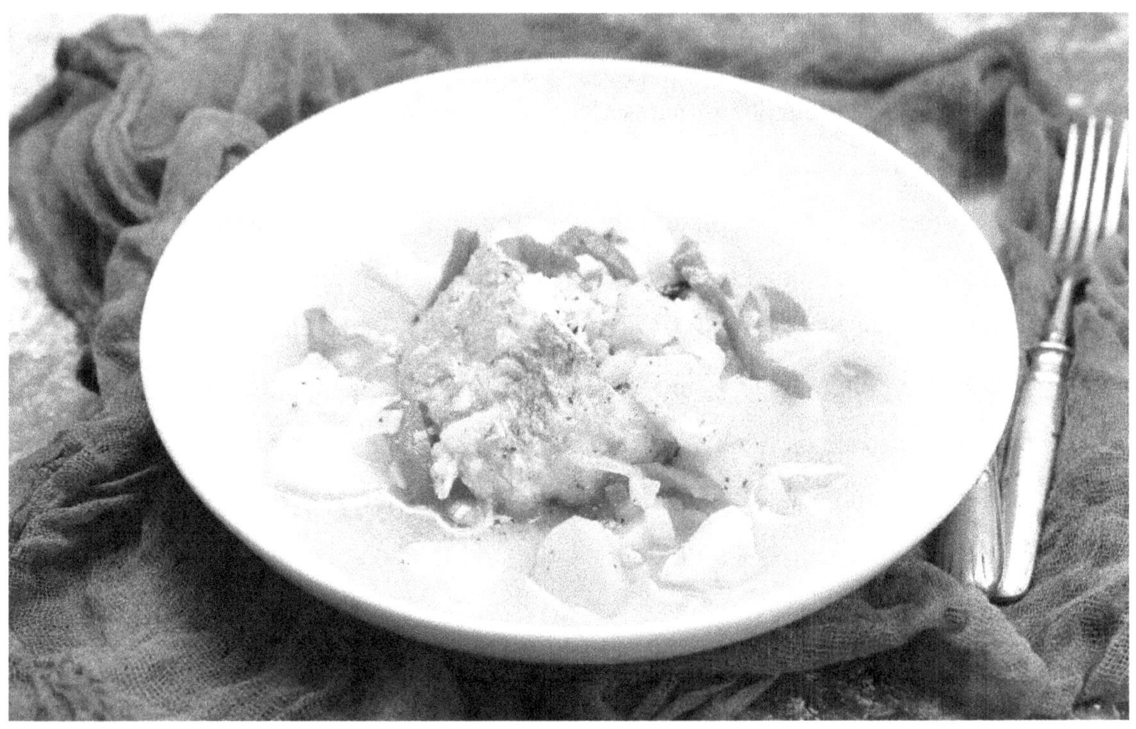

\No crustaceans added, just fish in a sumptuous broth. It is a quick meal to make you feel refreshed.

Prep Time: 15 mins

Cook Time: 38 mins

Serves: 4 to 6

Ingredients:

- ¼ cup extra-virgin olive oil
- ⅔ cup finely chopped shallots, from about 3 shallots
- 3 cloves garlic, minced
- 1 cup white wine
- 1 (28 oz) can crushed tomatoes
- 2 cups water
- 2 tsp sugar
- ½ tsp crushed red pepper flakes
- ½ tsp dried oregano
- 7 sprigs fresh thyme, plus 1 tsp chopped fresh thyme
- Kosher salt and black pepper to taste
- 4 ½ lb. firm-fleshed fish filets, such as halibut, cod, snapper, salmon, etc., cut into 2-inch pieces
- 3 tbsp unsalted butter
- Chopped fresh Italian parsley, for garnish, optional

Instructions:

1. Heat the olive oil in a large pot over medium heat. Sauté the shallots for 2 minutes. Add the garlic and sauté for 1 minute or until both are tender. Pour in the wine and let it reduce by half.
2. Add the tomatoes, water, sugar, red pepper flakes, oregano, thyme sprigs, salt, and black pepper. Bring to a boil and then simmer covered for 25 minutes.
3. Nestle the fish in and cook for 7 to 10 minutes or until the fish is opaque. Gently stir the butter through, making sure not to break the fish and let the butter melt.
4. Dish the soup in bowls, garnished with the remaining thyme and parsley, if preferred, and serve.

11. Gingery Chicken Soup with Zoodles

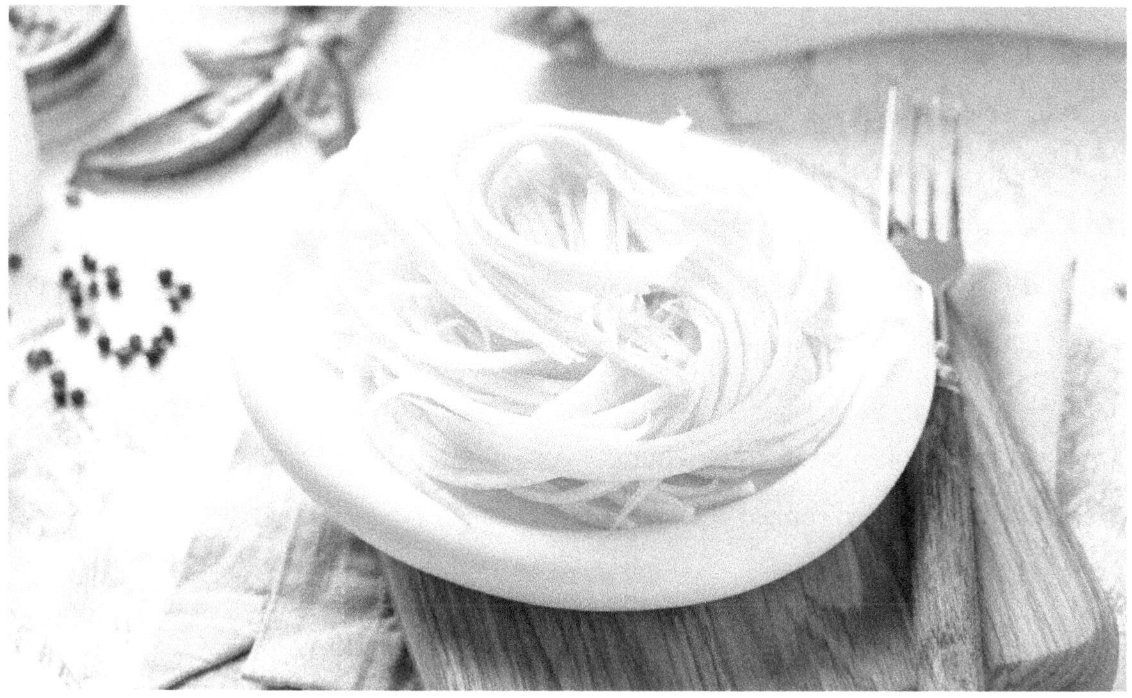

Caught a flu? Have a few spoonfuls of this slightly spicy-tangy soup and feel better.

Prep Time: 10 mins

Cook Time: 17 mins

Serves: 4

Ingredients:

- 1 tsp olive oil
- 1 ½ cups sliced carrots
- 2 celery stalks, sliced
- 3 green onions, sliced
- 2 cloves garlic
- 2 tbsp grated fresh ginger
- 2 tsp toasted sesame oil
- 3 to 5 tbsp soy sauce, low sodium
- 8 cups chicken broth, low sodium
- 2 cups shredded cooked chicken
- Salt to taste
- 1 large zucchini, spiralized into noodles
- Fresh cilantro leaves for garnish

Instructions:

1. Heat the oil in a large pot over medium heat. Sauté the carrots, celery, and green onions for 3 minutes or until tender. Stir in the garlic and ginger, and cook for 1 minute or until fragrant.
2. Add the sesame oil, soy sauce, and chicken broth; stir and bring to a boil. Add the chicken, stir, and simmer for 10 to 12 minutes or until the chicken warms through. Adjust the taste with salt as needed.
3. Stir in the zucchini noodles and cook for 1 minute. Serve the soup garnished with cilantro.

12. Dashi Broth with Mushrooms

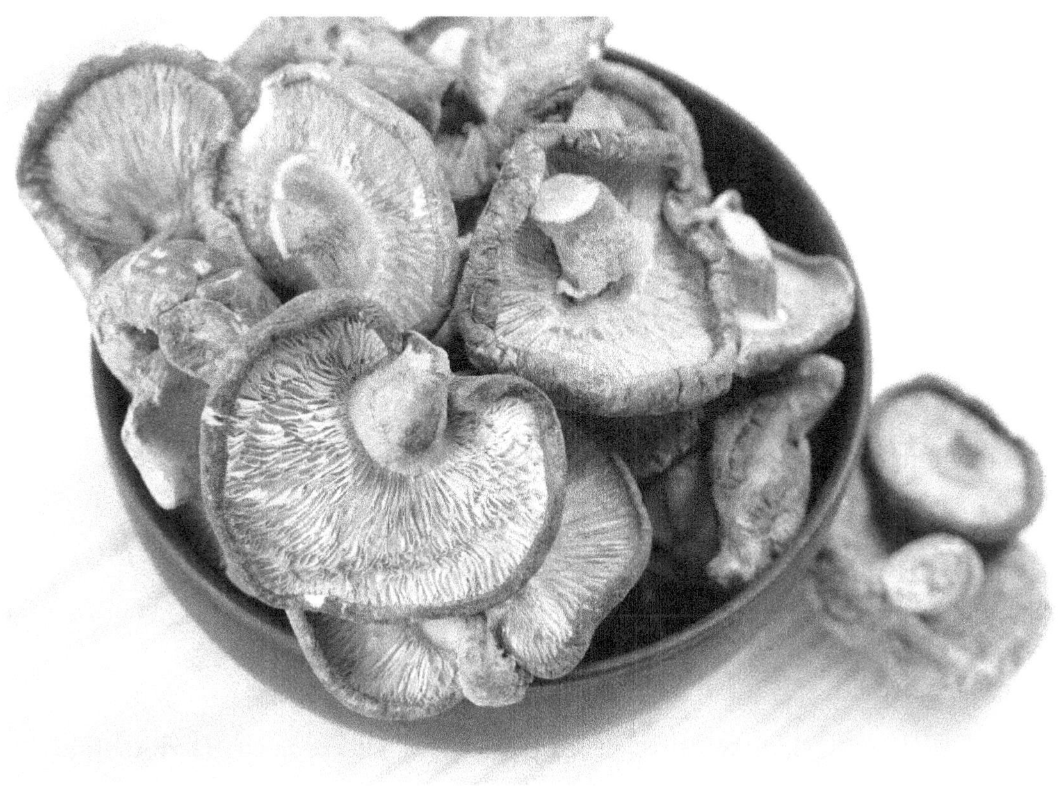

A treat without indulging in high-sugar foods. An abundance of mushrooms cooked in rich dashi broth that would warm your heart.

Prep Time: 20 mins

Cook Time: 12 hours

Serves: 4

Ingredients:

For the dashi:

- 7 cups water, divided
- 15 to 20 dried whole shiitake mushrooms, cleaned
- 1 (4×4-inch) piece kombu

For the soup:

- 8 shiitake mushrooms, stemmed, cut to 1 ½-inch pieces if larger
- 12 medium cremini mushrooms, cut to 1 ½-inch pieces if larger
- Reserved shiitake mushrooms from dashi, cut in half if large
- 2 tbsp olive or coconut oil, plus extra for coating
- 2 tsp + 3 tbsp soy sauce, divided
- 8 oz rice noodles
- 4 to 6 scallions, white and light green parts thinly sliced or chopped, dark green parts roughly sliced
- 1 ½ tbsp miso paste

Instructions:

For the dashi broth:

1. Add 3 cups of water and the mushrooms to a large pot. Weigh the mushrooms down with a heavy glass bowl and let them soak for 8 to 12 hours.
2. Remove the bowl, squeeze the liquid from the mushrooms into the broth, and reserve the mushrooms for the soup. Strain the broth through a fine mesh sieve lined with paper towels.
3. Heat the remaining 4 cups of water and kombu in a large pot. Just before the water boils, remove and discard the kombu. Add the mushroom liquid and turn the heat off.

For the soup:

1. Preheat the oven to 425°F.
2. Toss the mushrooms with oil and 2 tbsp of soy sauce. Spread them on a baking sheet and bake for 25 minutes or until the mushrooms are tender.
3. Cook the rice noodles according to the package's instructions. Drain and toss the noodles with a little oil to prevent them from sticking to each other.
4. Add the white and light green scallions to the dashi broth and bring to a simmer over low heat. Mix ¼ cup of the broth and miso paste in a bowl. Pour the mixture into the broth. Stir in the remaining soy sauce and keep warm.
5. Divide the noodles between serving bowls, add roasted mushrooms, and the deep green scallions. Add dashi broth to cover. Serve immediately.

13. Kimchi Tofu Stew

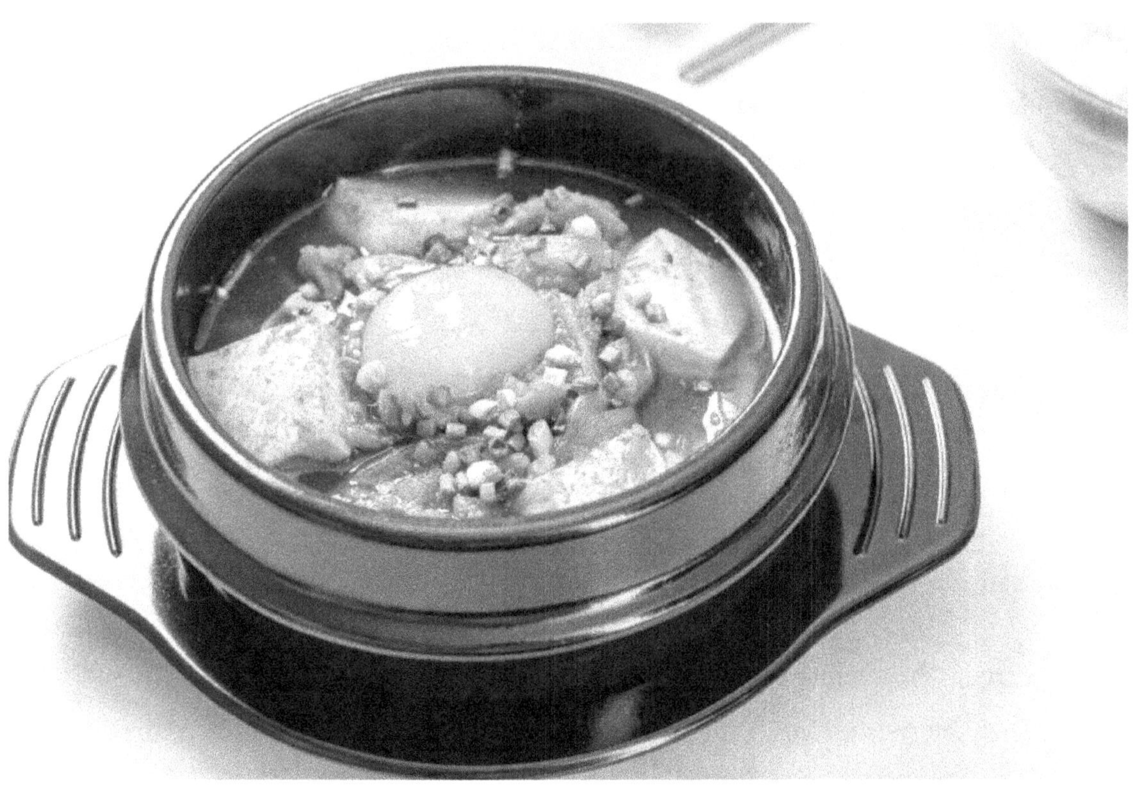

A colorful and loaded way to enjoy some probiotics with a spicy kick.

Prep Time: 10 mins

Cook Time: 20 mins

Serves: 4

Ingredients:

- 1 tbsp vegetable oil
- 4 garlic cloves, sliced
- 6 scallions, white and pale-green parts chopped, dark-green parts thinly sliced for garnish
- 1 (1-inch) piece ginger, peeled, finely chopped
- 4 cups chicken broth, low-sodium
- 3 tbsp soy sauce
- ½ cup kimchi
- 1 small daikon radish, peeled and sliced
- ¼ block firm silken tofu
- ½ cup kimchi

Instructions:

1. Heat the oil in a large pot over medium heat. Sauté the garlic, white and pale-green scallions, and ginger for 3 minutes or until fragrant. Add the broth, soy sauce, and gochujang; stir well. Add the daikon radish and simmer over low heat for 15 to 20 minutes or until tender.
2. Add the tofu and kimchi; simmer until the tofu warms through. Serve in bowls garnished with the deep green scallions.

14. Fig Goat Cheese Tartlets

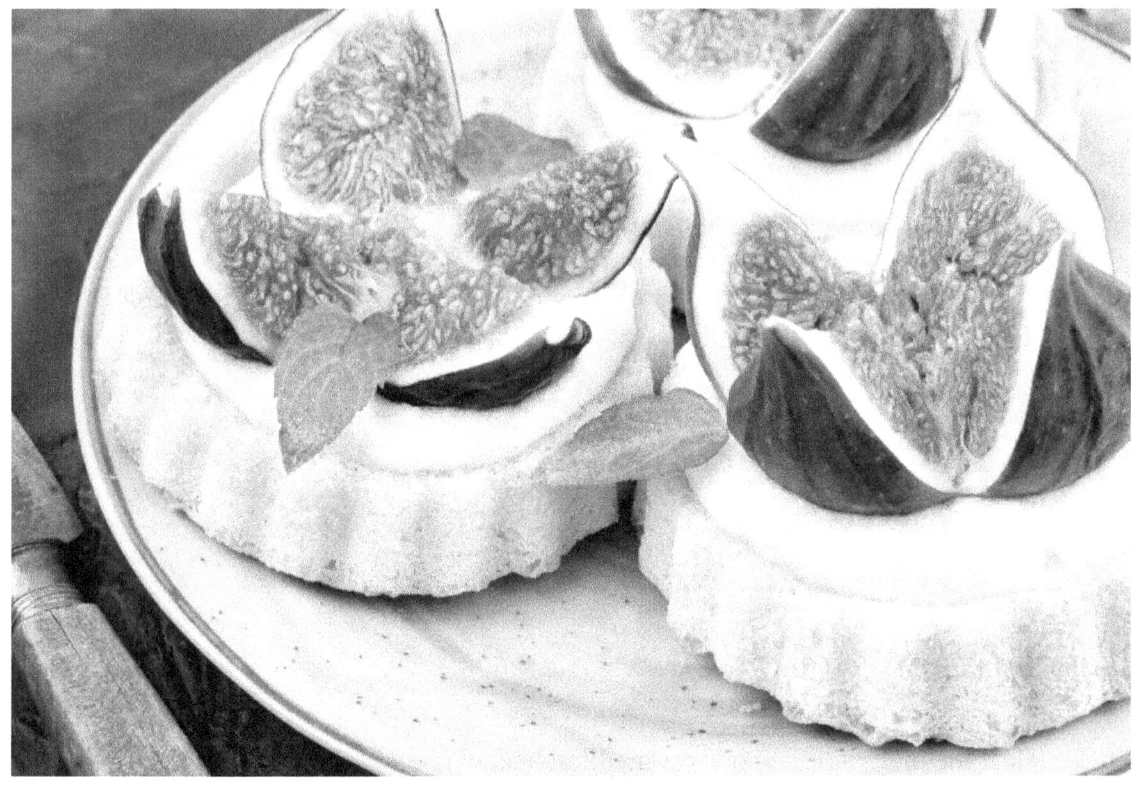

Healthy, crunchy, and hearty to satisfy your sugar cravings in a healthy way.

Prep Time: 10 mins

Cook Time: 10 mins

Makes: 16 pieces

Ingredients:

- 16 phyllo shells
- 4 oz soft goat cheese
- 4 figs, quartered
- 4 slices prosciutto, torn into 16 pieces
- Fresh thyme for garnish

Instructions:

1. Preheat the oven to 350°F.
2. Cut each pastry sheet into 4 pieces. Arrange the phyllo shells on a baking sheet. Spoon the goat cheese into shells, place 1 fig quarter on each, and a piece of prosciutto.
3. Bake for 7 to 10 minutes or until the shells are golden and crispy. Remove from the oven and garnish with thyme. Serve warm.

15. Chicken Meatballs, Green Beans, and Basil in Tomato Broth

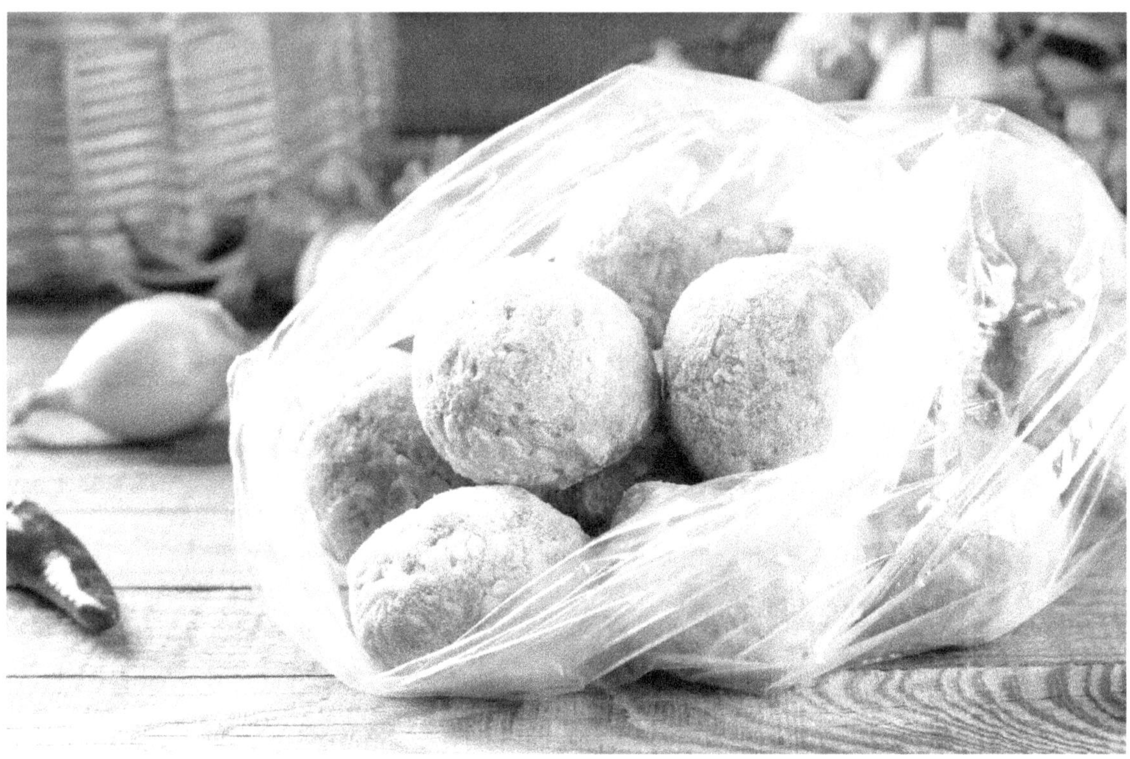

Frozen meatballs are used to help destress you while creating a light, rich, and satisfying tomato-basil soup.

Prep Time: 15 mins

Cook Time: 40 mins

Serves: 4

Ingredients:

- ¼ cup extra-virgin olive oil, divided
- 1 medium yellow onion, chopped
- ⅓ cup chopped carrots
- 4 garlic cloves, minced
- 2½ lb. roma tomatoes, halved
- 1 tsp thyme leaves
- Kosher salt and black pepper to taste
- 3 cups vegetable broth
- 12 oz frozen chicken meatballs
- 1 cup green beans, trimmed and cut into thirds
- 1 tbsp fresh lemon juice
- 1 loose-packed cup basil leaves, more for garnish

Instructions:

1. Heat the olive oil in a large pot over medium heat. Sauté the onion and carrots for 3 minutes or until tender. Stir in the garlic and cook for 1 minute or until fragrant. Add the tomatoes and season with salt and black pepper. Bring to a boil and simmer over low heat for 20 to 25 minutes or until the tomatoes are soft and breaking up.
2. Fetch out half of the tomatoes and purée the soup with an immersion blender. Stir the tomatoes back into the soup and add the meatballs; cook for 8 minutes. Stir in the green beans and cook for 2 to 3 more minutes or until tender and the meatballs are cooked through.
3. Turn the heat off and stir in the lemon juice, thyme, and basil. Serve warm.

16. Tomato, Bean, and Kale Soup

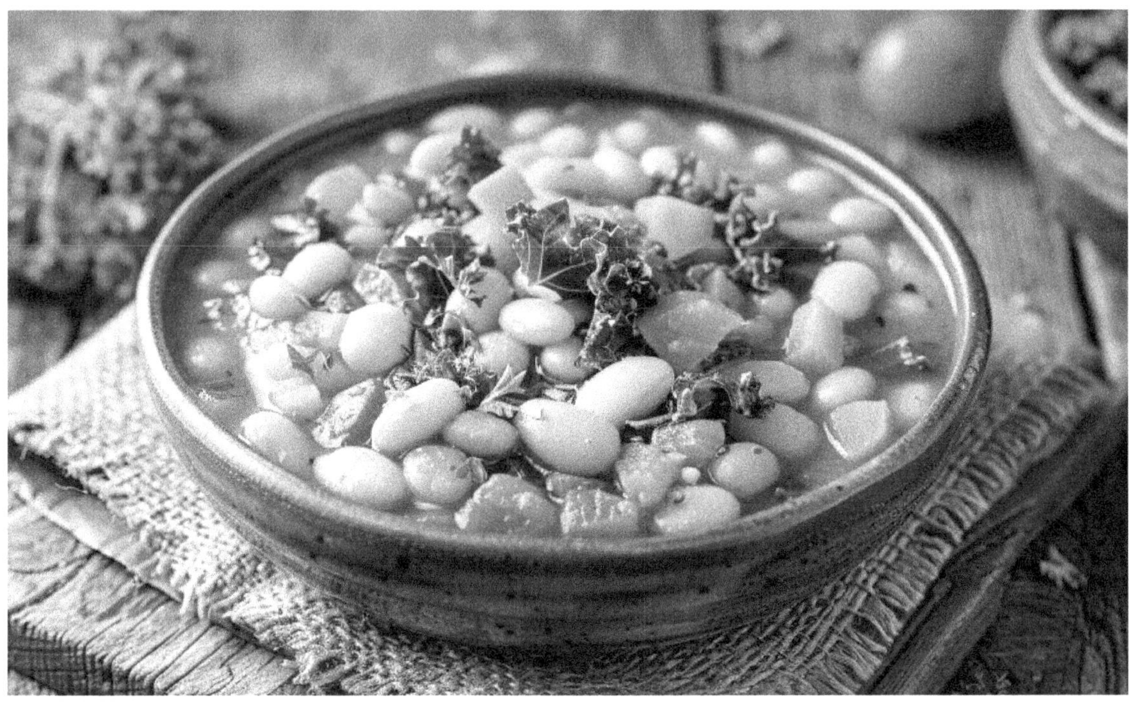

Use whatever white beans you like for a tomato-rich soup that will calm you after a long day.

Prep Time: 15 mins

Cook Time: 30 mins

Serves: 4

Ingredients:

- 1 tbsp olive oil
- 2 tbsp unsalted butter
- 1 large yellow or sweet onion, minced
- ½ tbsp fresh garlic, crushed
- ¼ tsp dried oregano
- ¼ tsp dried thyme
- 2 (14.5 oz) cans fire-roasted diced tomatoes
- 4 cups chicken or vegetable stock
- ¼ cup dry red wine
- Kosher salt and black pepper to taste
- 2 (15 oz) cans cooked white beans, drained but not rinsed
- 2 cups loosely-packed kale, rough stems removed and roughly chopped

Instructions:

1. Heat the olive oil and butter in a large pot over medium heat. Sauté the onion for 3 minutes, the garlic for 1 minute, and the oregano and thyme for 1 minute or until everything is tender and fragrant.
2. Add the tomatoes, stock, red wine, salt, and black pepper. Bring to a boil and simmer covered for 10 to 15 minutes.
3. Stir in the beans and cook for 5 minutes or until warmed through. Add the kale and cook for 2 to 3 minutes or until wilted. Adjust the rate with salt and black pepper. Serve warm.

17. Fresh Tomato and Basil Pasta

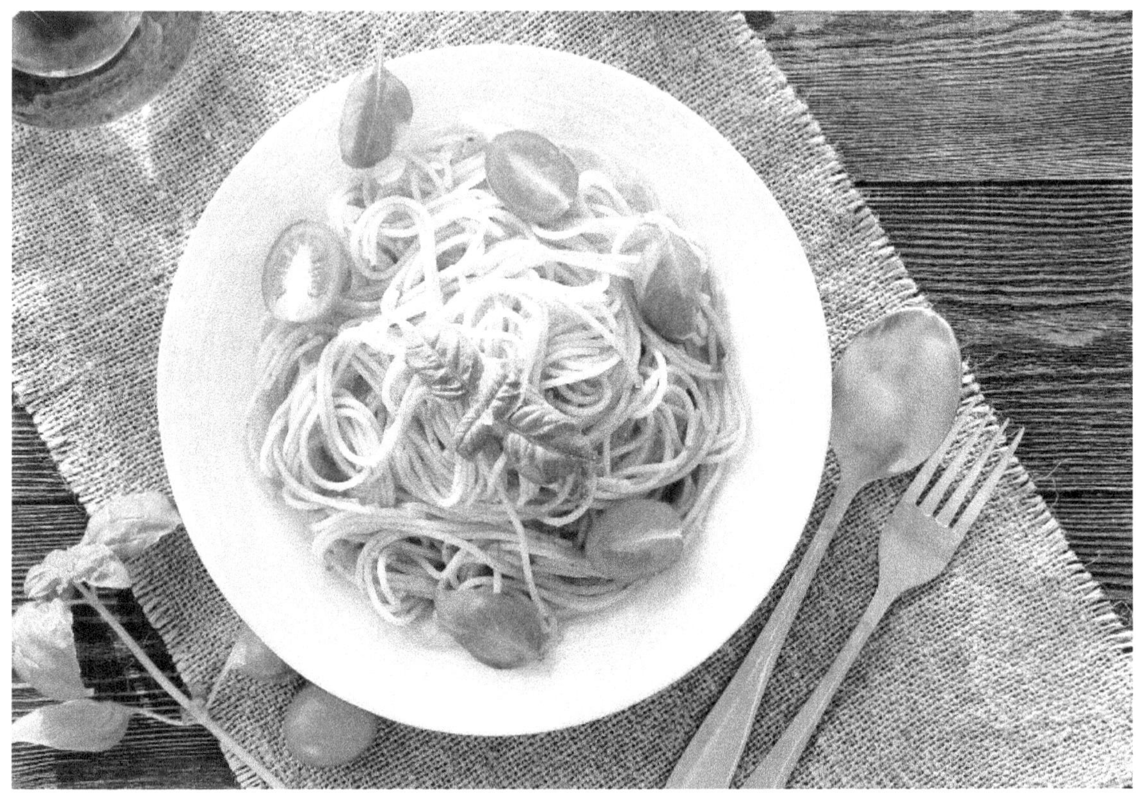

An 8-minute meal to quickly stop those hunger pangs from getting you irritated.

Prep Time: 10 mins

Cook Time: 8 mins

Serves: 4

Ingredients:

- 4 to 6 ripe tomatoes, chopped
- ⅓ cup basil leaves, stems removed, chopped
- 5 tbsp extra-virgin olive oil
- 2 tsp fresh lemon juice
- Kosher salt and black pepper to taste
- 1 lb. spaghetti, linguine, or fettuccine pasta
- ½ cup freshly grated Parmesan cheese

Instructions:

1. Toss the tomatoes, basil, olive oil, lemon juice, salt, and black pepper in a bowl. Set aside to marinate.
2. Cook the pasta according to the package's guide. Drain and return the pasta to the pot. Toss in the tomato mixture.
3. Serve immediately topped with Parmesan cheese.

18. Broiled Red Snapper with Za'atar Salsa Verde

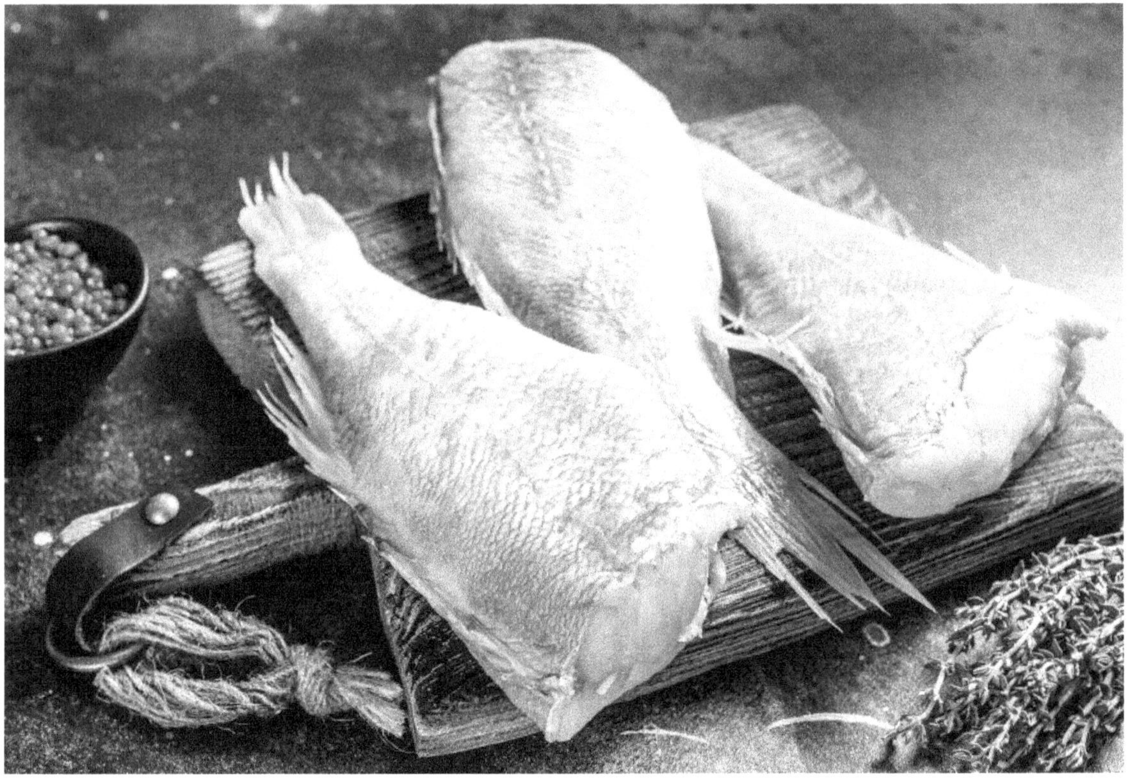

Paired with sautéed green beans would make for a light, green, and enriching meal.

Prep Time: 30 mins

Cook Time: 18 mins

Serves: 4

Ingredients:

- 4 (6 oz) skin-on, boneless red snapper filets, patted dry
- ⅓ cup finely chopped parsley
- 2 tbsp pine nuts
- ½ tsp ground coriander
- 4 tbsp plus ½ cup olive oil
- ⅓ cup finely chopped cilantro
- 1 garlic clove, finely grated
- 1½ tsp za'atar
- ¼ tsp crushed red pepper flakes
- 1 tbsp fresh lemon juice
- 2 tbsp finely chopped pickled banana peppers
- Kosher salt to taste

Instructions:

1. Toast the pine nuts in a skillet over medium heat for 3 minutes. Cool completely and coarsely chop them. Set aside.
2. Preheat the broiler.
3. Season the snapper with salt and coriander. Drizzle 2 tbsp of olive oil on a baking sheet, lay in the fish, skin side down, and drizzle with 2 tbsp olive oil. Broil for 8 to 10 minutes or until the skin is crisp and browned. Rest the fish out of the broiler for 5 minutes.
4. Mix the remaining ingredients and pine nuts in a bowl. Season with salt.
5. Plate the fish, skin side up, and spoon on the za'atar mixture. Serve right away.

19. Seasonal Chicken Soup

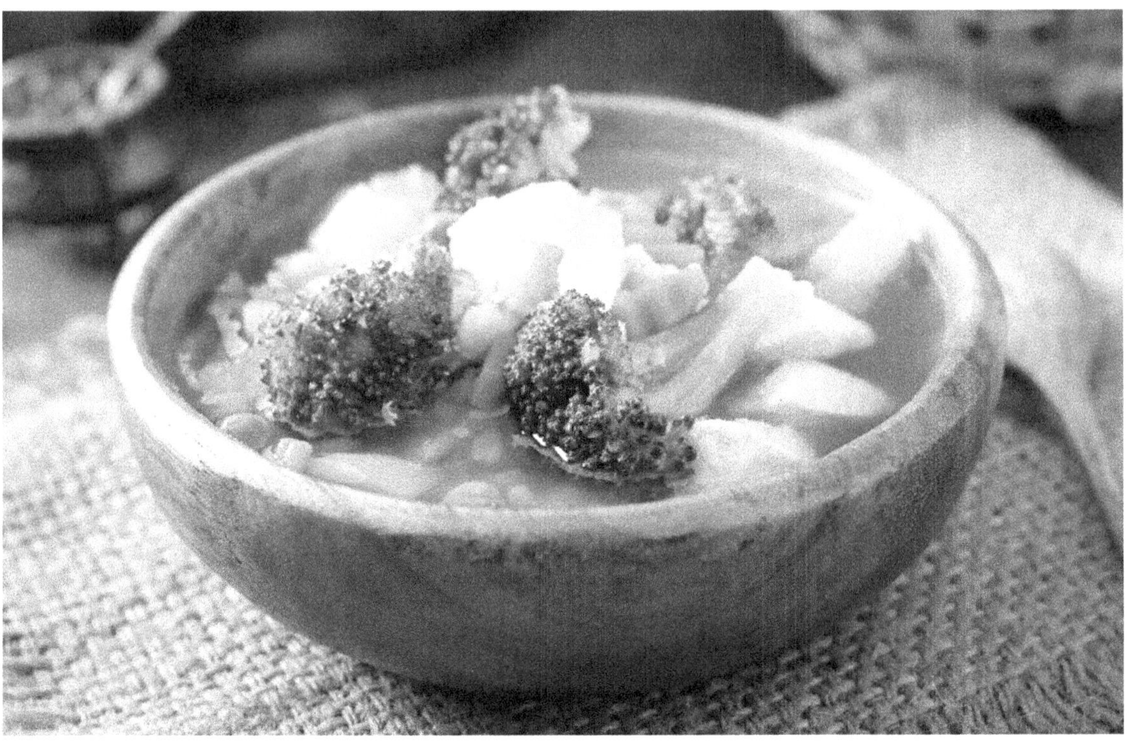

Perfect to drive away the cold, you can opt chicken out, and still enjoy a warm, flavorful soup.

Prep Time: 20 mins

Cook Time: 20 mins

Serves: 4

Ingredients:

- 1 tbsp olive oil
- 1 yellow onion, peeled and chopped
- 2 carrots, sliced in ¼-inch slices
- 2 celery stalks, sliced in ¼-inch slices
- 4 cups homemade chicken stock
- 2 cups shredded cooked chicken (exclude for a meatless option)
- 1 tbsp fresh parsley leaves
- 1 tbsp chopped greens from a green onion
- ¼ tsp ground sage and thyme
- A small pinch of cayenne pepper
- Kosher salt and black pepper to taste

Instructions:

1. Heat the olive oil in a large pot over medium heat. Next, sauté the onion, carrots, and celery for 3 minutes or until tender.
2. Pour in the chicken stock and bring to a boil. Add the chicken (if using), parsley, green onions, sage and thyme, and cayenne pepper. Simmer covered for 10 to 15 minutes or until heated through. Adjust the taste with salt and black pepper.
3. Serve warm.

20. Salmon Poke on Greens and Peas

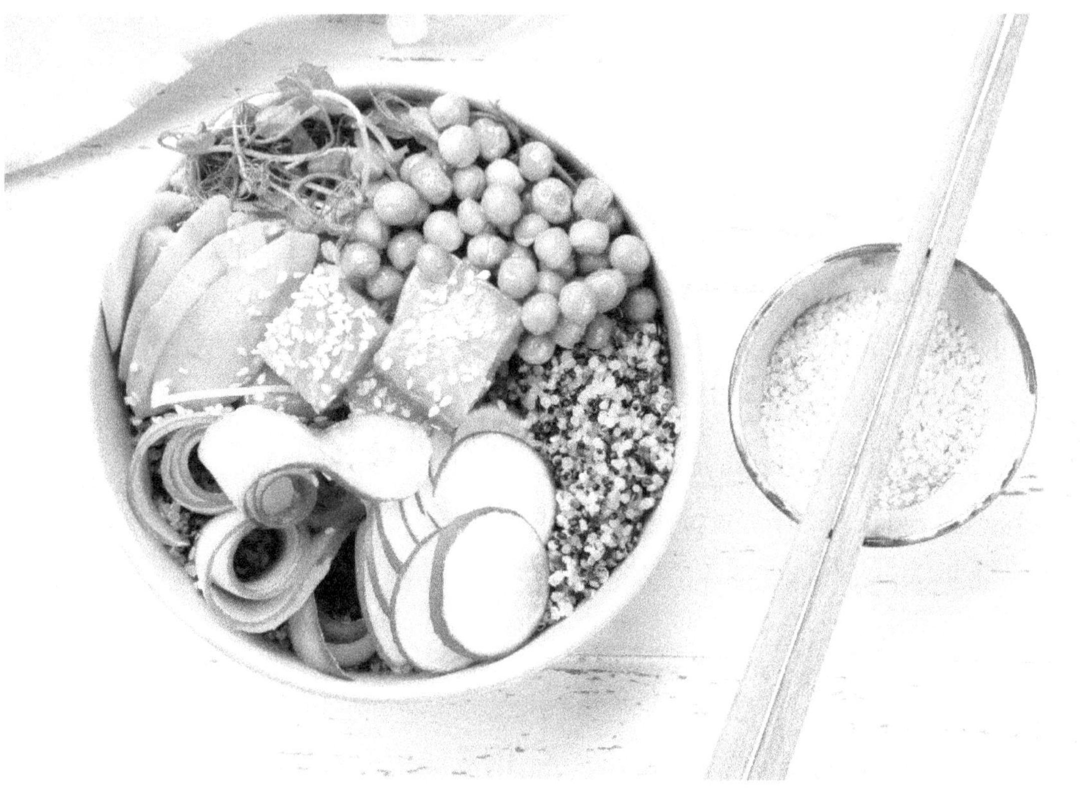

A salad that would make you feel better of yourself again. The dressing does a good number to the tastiness of the entire dish.

Prep Time: 20 mins

Serves: 4

Ingredients:

- 2 Persian cucumbers, thinly sliced
- Kosher salt
- 1 tsp caster sugar
- 2 tbsp unseasoned rice vinegar, divided
- ½ tsp finely grated peeled ginger
- 3 tbsp white or dark soy sauce
- 1 ½ tbsp mirin
- 1 ½ tbsp fresh grapefruit juice
- 1 tsp fresh lemon juice
- 1 scallion, finely chopped
- 5 heads little gem lettuce, cores removed and leaves separated
- 12 oz salmon poke
- 1 avocado, cut into ½-inch pieces
- ¼ cup cooked peas

Instructions:

1. Put the cucumbers in a strainer. Sprinkle them with salt and let sit for 10 minutes. Meanwhile, mix the sugar, vinegar, and ginger in a bowl. Massage the liquid off the cucumber, add it to the sugar mixture and toss well. Set aside.

2. Whisk the soy sauce, mirin, grapefruit juice, lemon juice, and scallion in a bowl. Add 3 tbsp of the mixture to another bowl; toss the salmon with this mixture. Toss the smaller amount with the lettuce.

3. Arrange the lettuce on a platter and top with the pickled cucumber, salmon, avocado, and peas. Serve right away.

21. Cream of Cashew Pea Soup

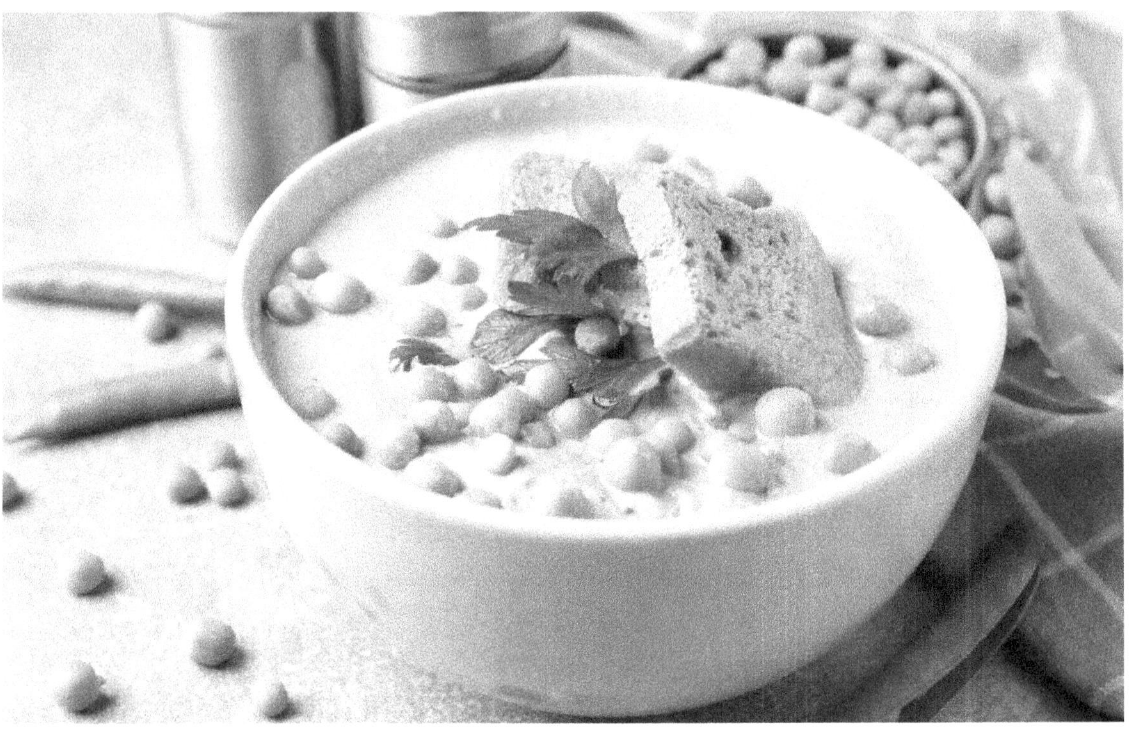

Peas and cashews are a creamy delicious combo, making this soup feel like an embrace. Enjoy silky smooth swallows all through.

Prep Time: 10 mins

Cook Time: 15 mins

Serves: 4

Ingredients:

- 1 tbsp olive oil
- 1 yellow onion, chopped
- 5 stalks celery, chopped
- 4 large cloves garlic, minced
- 2 cups raw cashews, soaked overnight, drained, and rinsed
- 7 cups green peas, fresh or frozen
- 4 cups water
- Kosher salt to taste
- Sliced green onions for garnish

Instructions:

1. Heat the olive oil in a pot over medium heat. Sauté the onion and celery for 3 minutes. Add the garlic and sauté for 1 minute or until everything is tender and fragrant.
2. Add the cashews, peas, and water. Bring to a boil and simmer for 10 minutes or until the peas are soft. Purée the soup with an immersion blender until smooth. Season with salt.
3. Serve the soup in bowls garnished with green onions.

22. Chocolate Truffles

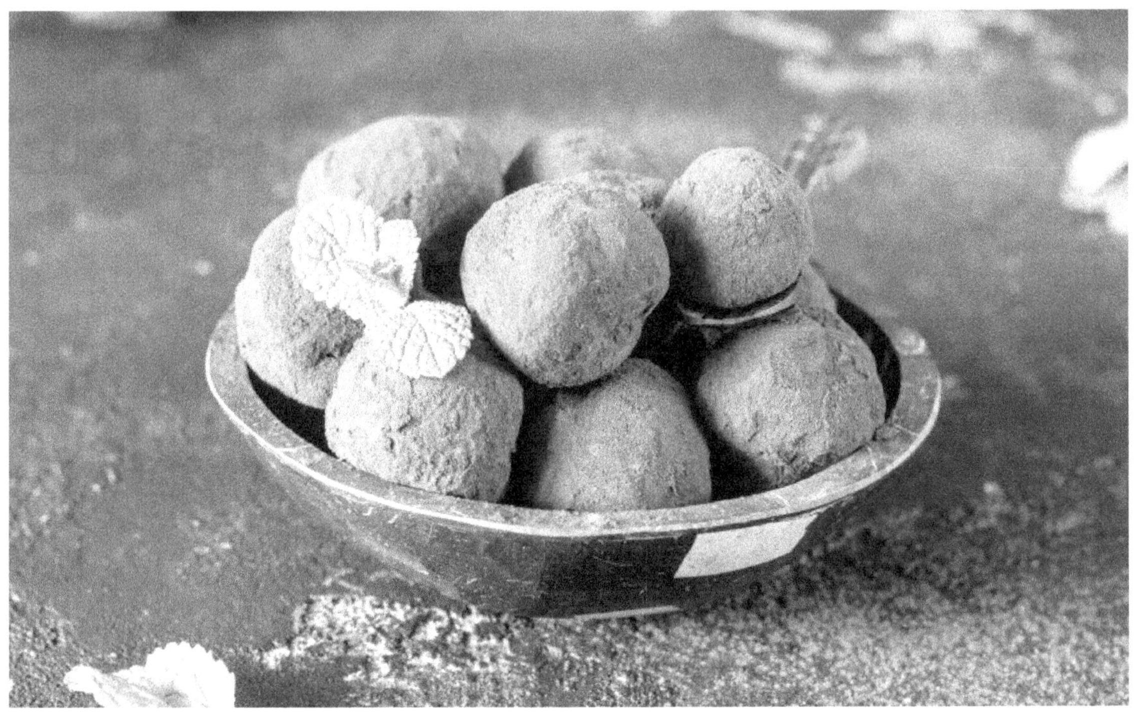

After a long day, a bite of one chocolate truffle is so rewarding.

Prep Time: 20 mins

Cook Time: 2 mins

Chill Time: 6 hours

Serves: 8

Ingredients:

- 10 oz dark chocolate, chopped
- 2 tbsp unsalted butter
- ½ cup heavy cream
- Cocoa powder for coating

Instructions:

1. Combine the chocolate, butter, and heavy cream in a safe microwave bowl. Microwave on high for 2 minutes, stirring at 30 seconds intervals.
2. Cover the bowl with a plate and let it stand for 5 minutes. After, stir the mixture until the chocolate is fully melted and smooth. Refrigerate covered for 6 hours - don't freeze. Also, refrigerate a serving plate or tray as well.
3. Roll 1 tbsp-size balls from the chilled chocolate mixture.
4. Roll the truffles in cocoa powder until well coated and place them on the chilled plate. Enjoy!

23. Coconut-Lime Energy Bites

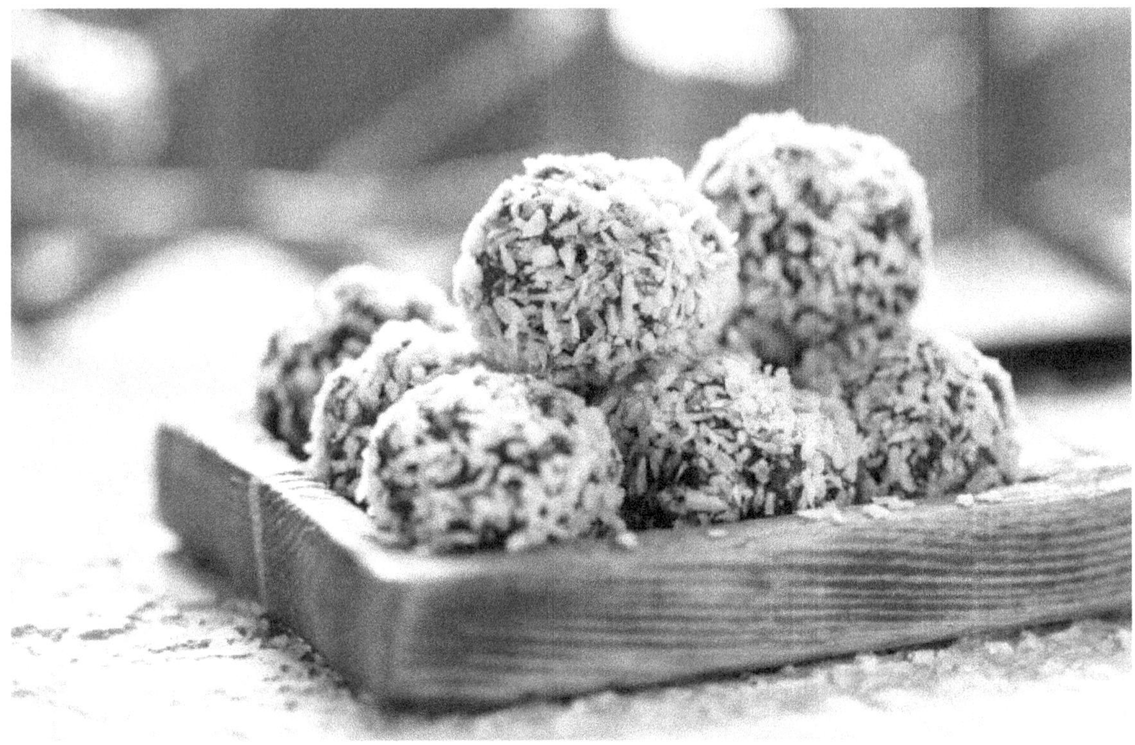

One perfect work companion to help motivate you through the day,

Prep Time: 15 mins

Serves: 4

Ingredients:

- 1 cup raw cashews
- 1 cup packed pitted soft dates
- ⅔ cup unsweetened fine coconut, plus extra for rolling
- 2 tbsp fresh lime juice
- 1 tsp grated fresh lime zest

Instructions:

1. Grind the cashews in a food processor until coarse and grainy. Add the dates and grind until a crumbly, sticky dough forms. Add the coconut, lime juice, and lime zest; grind until smooth and sticky.
2. Roll 1 tbsp-size balls from the mixture and roll each ball in coconut until well coated. Serve.

24. Mango-Yogurt Pudding

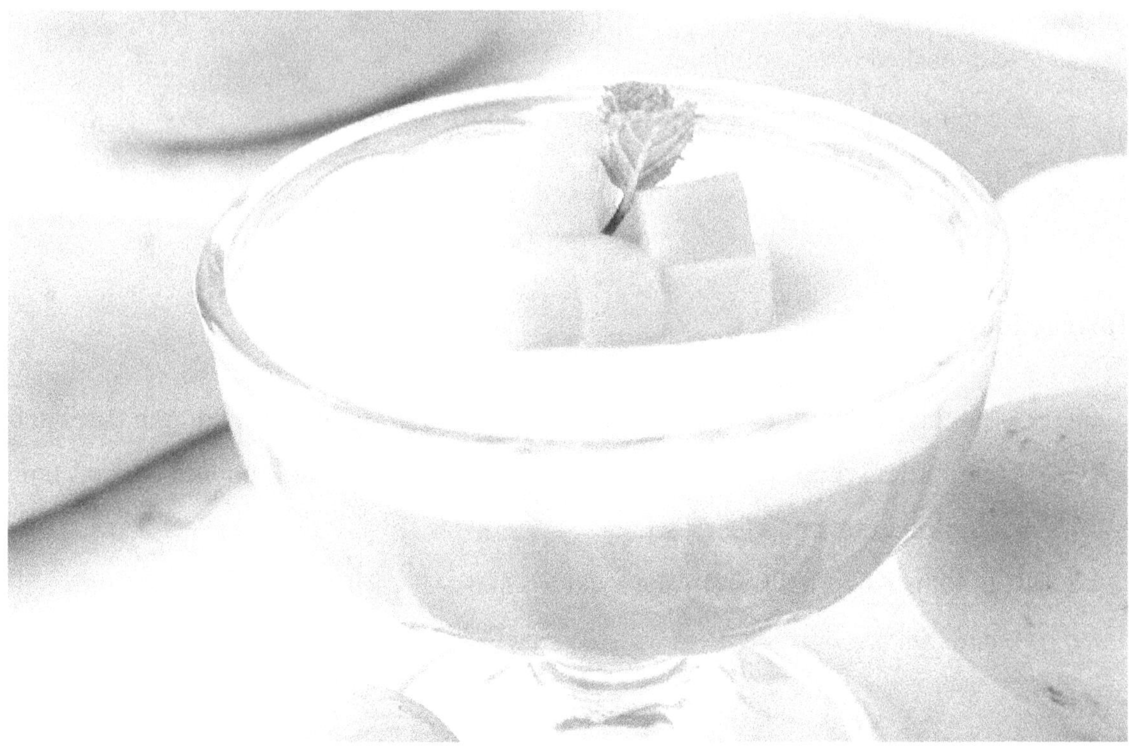

Take a chill on the balcony while enjoying this creamy fruit pudding to aid with some reflection.

Prep Time: 10 mins

Chill Time: 1 hour

Serves: 4

Ingredients:

- 1 cup full-fat coconut milk or other milk of choice
- 3 tbsp chia seeds
- 2 tbsp pure maple syrup, divided
- 1 ½ cups puréed mango
- ½ cup vanilla yogurt
- Chopped mango, chia seeds, and coconut flakes for garnish

Instructions:

1. Mix the coconut milk, chia seeds, and 1 tbsp maple syrup in a bowl. Cover and refrigerate for 1 hour.
2. When ready to serve, mix the mango purée, yogurt, and remaining maple syrup in a bowl.
3. Layer the chia pudding and mango mixture in serving glasses. Garnish with chopped mango, chia seeds, and coconut flakes. Serve.

25. Cherry Chocolate Marble Cake

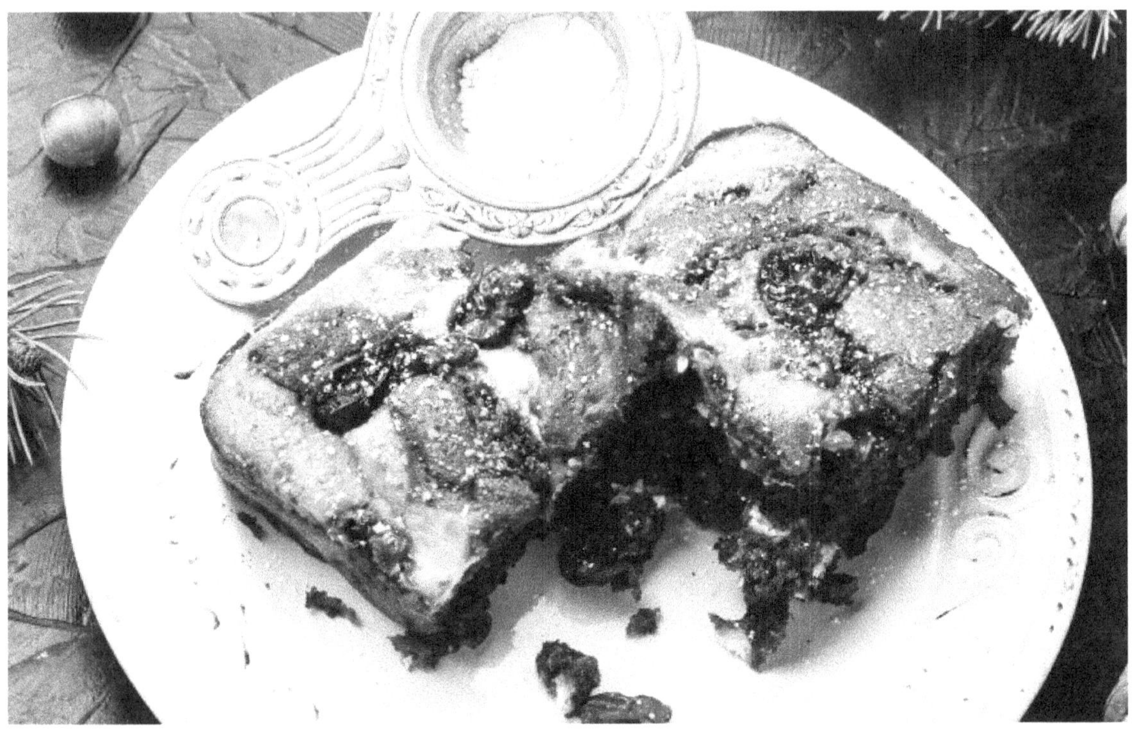

Cherry and chocolate are a beautiful combination in this cake. All you need is a slice to help make you feel whole again.

Prep Time: 20 mins

Cook Time: 1 hour 15 mins

Serves: 12

Ingredients:

- 1 cup butter, softened
- 2 cups granulated sugar
- 3 large eggs, room temperature
- 6 tbsp maraschino cherry juice
- 6 tbsp water
- 1 tsp almond extract
- 3 ¾ cups all-purpose flour
- 2 ¼ tsp baking soda
- ¾ tsp salt
- 1 ½ cups sour cream
- ¾ cup chopped walnuts, toasted
- ¾ cup chopped maraschino cherries, drained
- 3 oz unsweetened chocolate, melted

Instructions:

1. Preheat the oven to 350°F. Grease and flour a 10-inch fluted tube pan. Set aside.
2. Cream the butter and sugar in a bowl until light and fluffy. Whisk in 1 egg at a time until each addition is smooth. Add the cherry juice, water, and almond extract; whisk until smooth. Mix the flour, baking soda, and salt in a bowl. Alternate mixing the flour mixture and sour cream with the egg batter until smooth.
3. Divide the batter in half. In one portion, fold the walnuts and cherries. Mix the chocolate with the other portion until smooth. Spoon half of the cherry batter into the cake pan and top with half of the chocolate batter. Repeat the layers.
4. Bake for 1 ¼ hours or until baked through. Rest the cake in the pan for 15 minutes before transferring it to a wire rack to cool completely. Slice and serve.

26. Roasted Strawberry Sheet Cake

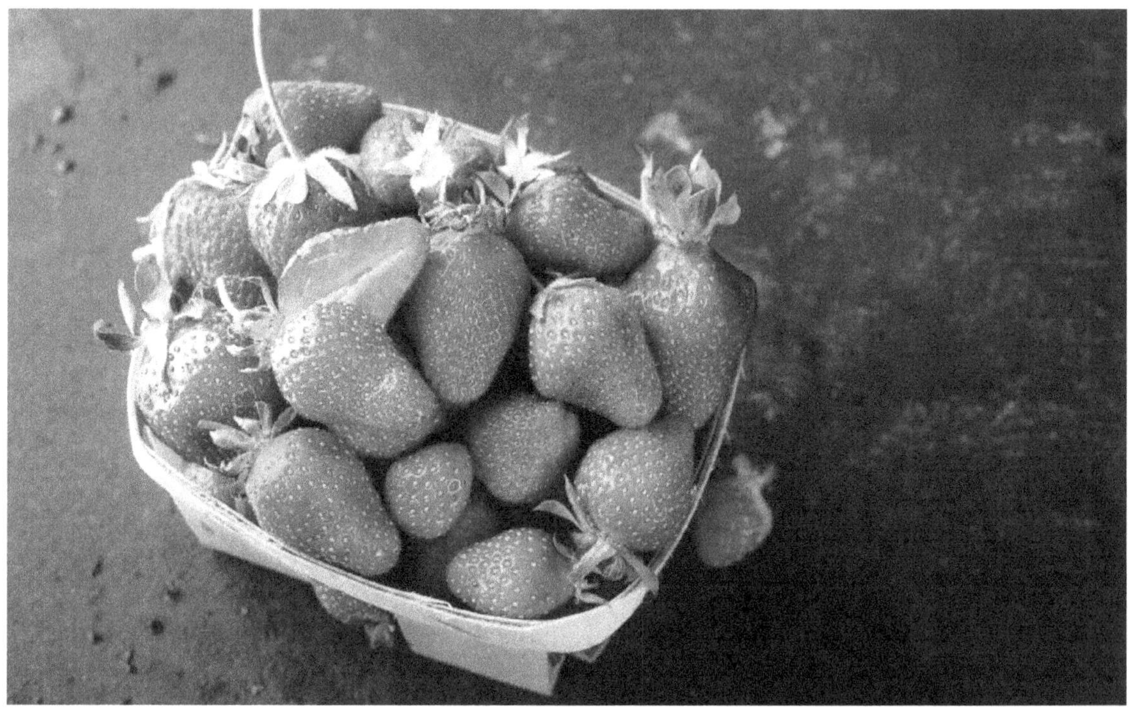

Keep squares of this roasted strawberry delight refrigerated and close by. Grab a piece whenever you like to help kick the stress away.

Prep Time: 30 mins

Cook Time: 75 mins

Serves: 24

Ingredients:

- 4 lb. halved fresh strawberries
- 2 cups granulated sugar, divided
- 1 cup butter, softened
- 2 large eggs, room temperature
- 2 tsp almond extract
- 3 cups all-purpose flour
- 3 tsp baking powder
- 2 tsp salt
- 1 cup 2% milk
- ¼ cup turbinado sugar

Instructions:

1. Preheat the oven to 350°F. Line 2 rimmed baking sheets with baking paper.
2. Add the strawberries to one baking sheet, sprinkle with ½ cup of granulated sugar, and toss to coat. Spread out evenly and bake for 35 to 40 minutes or until tender.
3. Meanwhile, cream the butter and remaining granulated sugar in a bowl until light and fluffy. Whisk in 1 egg at a time until each addition is smooth. Whisk in the almond extract until smooth. Mix the flour, baking powder, and salt in a bowl. Alternate mixing the flour mixture and milk with the egg batter - the batter may look curdled, which is fine).
4. Pour the batter onto the clean baking sheet and spread 3 cups of the roasted strawberries on top (reserve the remaining strawberries for serving). Sprinkle with turbinado sugar and bake for 30 to 35 minutes or until the batter bakes through. Cool the cake completely in the pan on a wire rack. Cut into squares and serve with the reserved strawberries.

27. Chocolate Chip Cookie Sticks

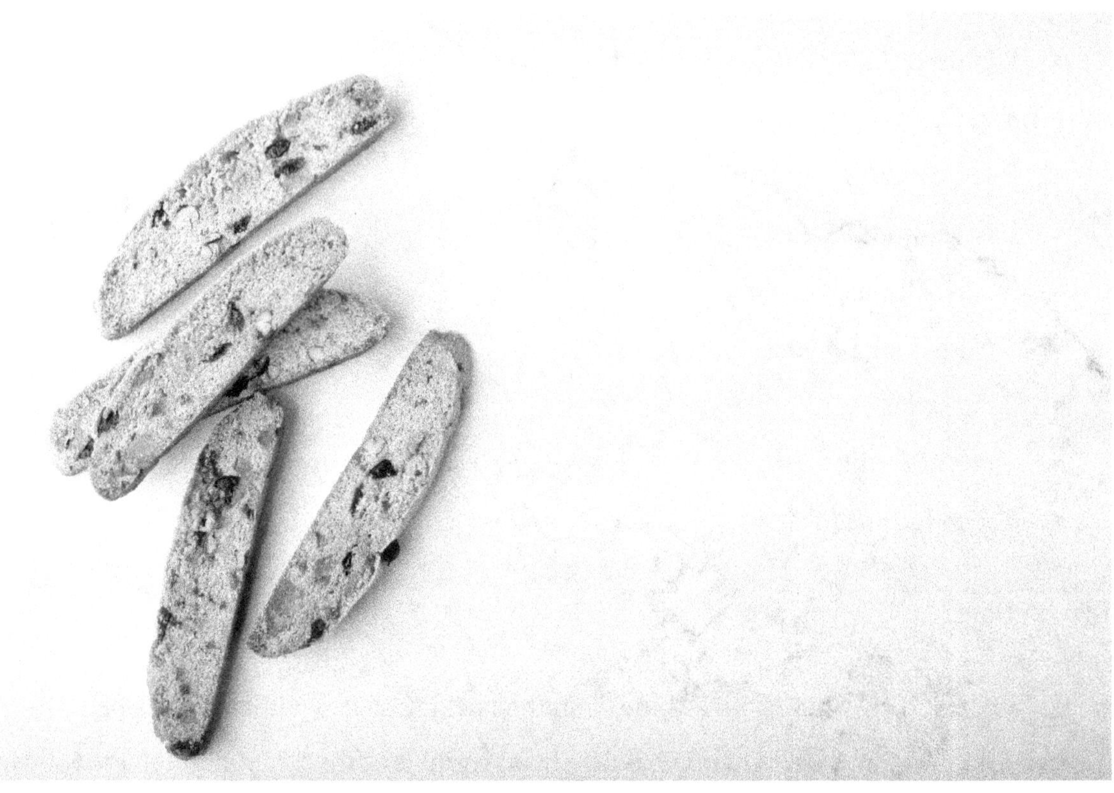

Creating these cookies is a relieving way to destress and have a moment to yourself particularly when pressing the dough into the baking sheet before baking.

Prep Time: 30 mins

Cook Time: 10 mins

Makes: 36 strips

Ingredients:

- ½ cup canola oil
- ½ cup packed brown sugar
- ½ cup granulated sugar
- 1 large egg, room temperature
- 1 tsp vanilla extract
- 1 ½ cups all-purpose flour
- ½ tsp baking soda
- ½ tsp salt
- 1 cup semisweet chocolate chips
- ½ cup chopped walnuts

Instructions:

1. Preheat the oven to 375°F. Grease a rimmed baking sheet with oil.
2. Whisk the oil, both sugar types, egg, and vanilla in a bowl until smooth. Mix the flour, baking soda, and salt in a bowl; gradually whisk with the egg mixture until smooth dough forms. Spread and fit the dough on the baking sheet, forming a rectangle. Sprinkle the chocolate chips and walnuts on top.
3. Bake for 6 to 10 minutes or until baked through and crispy to your liking. Cool for 5 minutes. Slice into 36 strips and cool on a wire rack.

28. Banana Skillet Upside-Down Cake

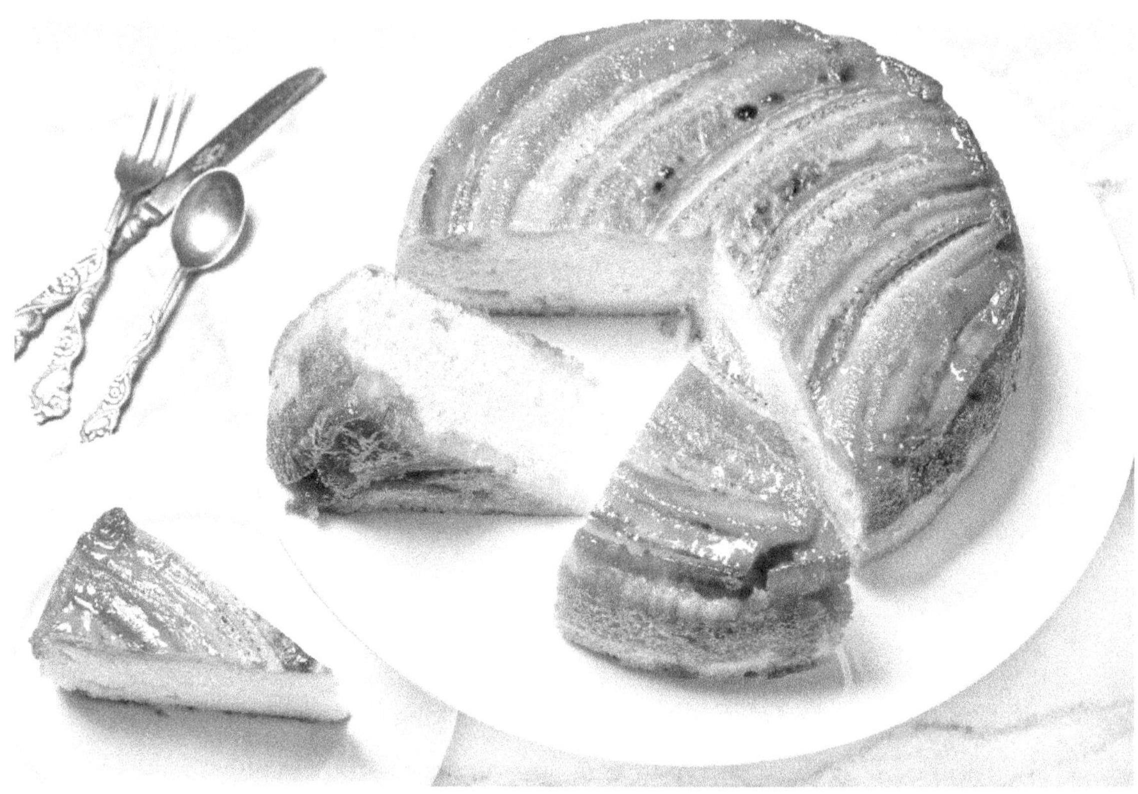

Create your twist of pineapple upside down cake as a fun project and enjoy a sweeter version with bananas.

Prep Time: 20 mins

Cook Time: 45 mins

Serves: 10

Ingredients:

- 1 (14 oz) package banana quick bread and muffin mix
- ½ cup chopped walnuts
- ¼ cup butter, cubed
- ¾ cup packed brown sugar
- 2 tbsp lemon juice
- 4 medium bananas, cut into ¼-inch slices
- 2 cups sweetened shredded coconut

Instructions:

1. Preheat the oven to 375°F.
2. Prepare the bread and muffin mix according to the package's guide. Fold in the walnuts. Set aside.
3. Melt the butter in a 10-inch ovenproof skillet over medium heat. Add the brown sugar and stir for 3 minutes or until dissolved. Stir in the lemon juice and cook for 2 to 3 minutes or until thickened. Turn the heat off and arrange the bananas on top in a single layer; sprinkle with coconut.
4. Spoon the prepared batter over the coconut and banana. Bake for 35 to 40 minutes or until dark golden brown and baked through.
5. Cool for 5 minutes in the skillet and invert it onto a large serving platter. Slice and serve.

29. Tiramisu Cookies

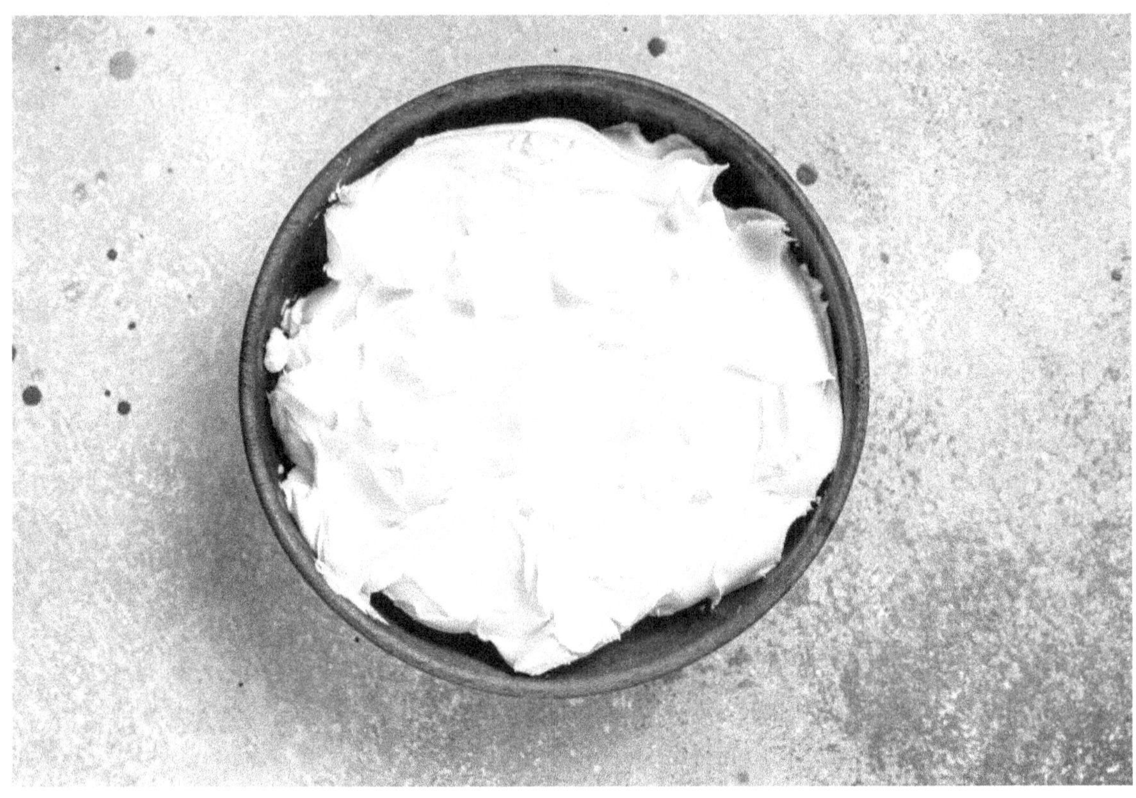

Deconstruct traditional tiramisu and enjoy a creative moment reassembling it into creamy cookies.

Prep Time: 15 mins

Cook Time: 14 mins

Makes: 18

Ingredients:

For the cookies:

- ¾ cup granulated sugar
- 1 cup butter, softened
- 2 large eggs, room temperature
- 1 tsp vanilla extract
- 1 tsp baking powder
- ½ tsp rum extract
- 2 ¼ cups all-purpose flour
- ¼ tsp salt

For the filling:

- 1 (8 oz) carton mascarpone cheese
- ¼ cup butter, softened
- 2 tsp instant coffee granules
- 1 tsp vanilla extract
- 3 cups confectioners' sugar
- Cocoa powder for dusting

Instructions:

For the cookies:

1. Preheat the oven to 350°F. Line a baking sheet with baking paper. Set aside.
2. Cream the butter and sugar in a bowl until light and fluffy. Next, whisk in 1 egg at a time until each addition is smooth. Mix in the vanilla and rum extracts until smooth. Mix the flour, baking soda, and salt in a bowl. Gradually whisk the mixture into the egg batter until smooth.
3. Drop 2-tbsp sized dough pieces at intervals on the baking sheet. Dip the bottom of a glass in confectioner's sugar and slightly flatten the dough pieces. Bake for 12 to 14 minutes or until the edges slightly brown. Cool the cookies completely on a wire rack.

For the filling:

1. Cream the mascarpone cheese and butter in a bowl until smooth. In a small bowl, dissolve the instant coffee granules with vanilla and whisk into the cheese mixture. Gradually mix in the confectioner's sugar until smooth. Pipe or spread the filling onto half of the flatter side of the cookies. Cover with the remaining cookies. Dust the cookies with cocoa powder. Enjoy and store extras in the refrigerator.

30. Chocolate Swirl Cheesecake

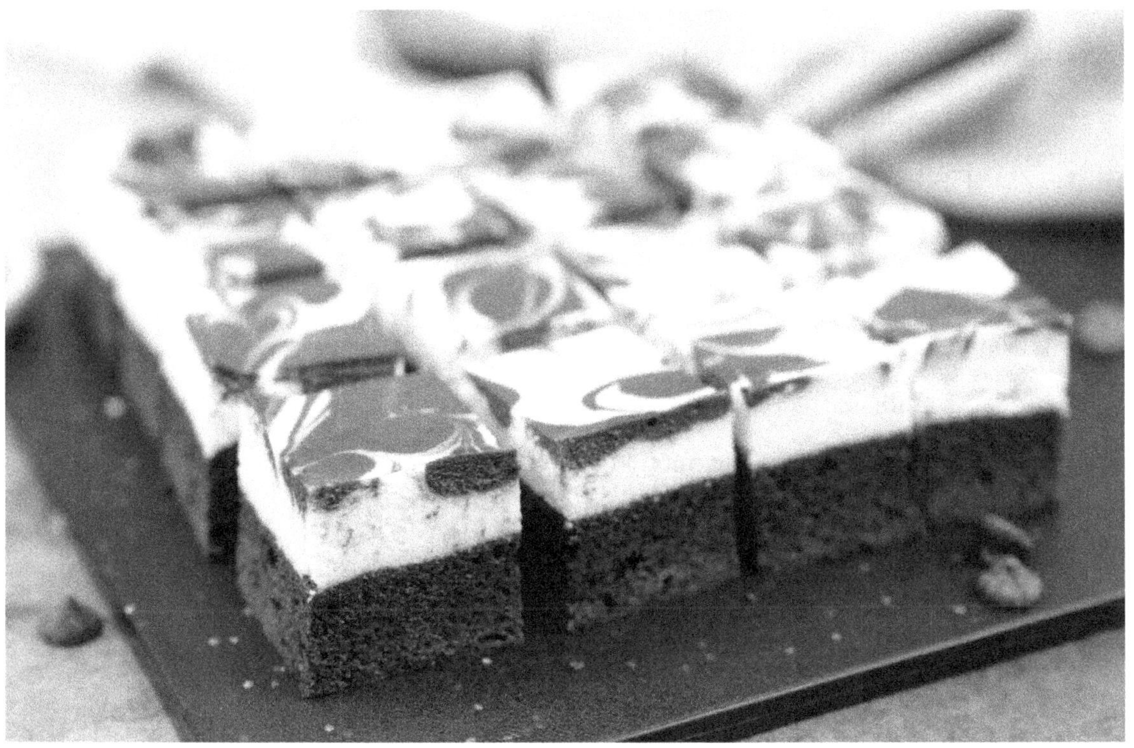

The fun is in swirling the chocolate through the creamy batter before baking. Take the time to unwind while playing through the batter and creating an amazing marble pattern.

Prep Time: 1 hour 20 mins

Cook Time: 40 mins

Chill Time: 1 hour + overnight chilling

Serves: 12

Ingredients:

- 2 cups 2% cottage cheese, well-strained
- 1 cup crushed chocolate wafers
- 1(8 oz) package cream cheese, cubed
- ½ cup granulated sugar
- A pinch of salt
- 2 large eggs, lightly beaten
- 1 large egg white
- 1 tbsp vanilla extract
- 2 oz bittersweet chocolate, melted and cooled
- Boiling water, as needed

Instructions:

1. Refrigerate the strained cottage cheese for 1 hour.

2. Double line a 9-inch springform pan with heavy-duty foil. Wrap foil around the pan too. Grease inside the pan with cooking spray. Press the crushed wafers onto the bottom and 1-inch side up of the pan. Place on a rimmed baking sheet.

3. Preheat the oven to 350°F.

4. Add the cottage cheese to a food processor and process until smooth. Add the cream cheese, sugar, and salt; process until smooth. Pour the mixture into a bowl and whisk in the eggs, egg white, and vanilla until smooth. Add 1 cup of batter to another bowl and stir in the chocolate. Pour the plain batter onto the wafer crust and drop spoonfuls of the chocolate batter over the top. Use a skewer to swirl the chocolate batter through for a marble-like pattern.

5. Pour 1-inch of boiling water on the baking sheet. Carefully transfer to the oven with the cake pan and bake for 40 minutes or until the top appears dull. Slightly open the oven and cool the cheesecake in it for 30 minutes.

6. Remove the foil and cool on a wire rack for 30 minutes. Transfer the pan to the refrigerator, cover, and chill overnight or until completely cooled.

7. Remove the pan's rim from the cheesecake when ready to slice and serve.

Conclusion

We hope these recipes kick some joy within to get onto some creative, healthy, nourishing, and fun cooking.

With recipes ranging from easy to moderate makes, we desire that cooking them feels like art as you enjoy the wonderful colors, awesome tastes, and feel-good factor that they offer.

Also, be at ease to tweak the recipes to your desire - it's all about having fun at them to make you feel better.

Dear Reader

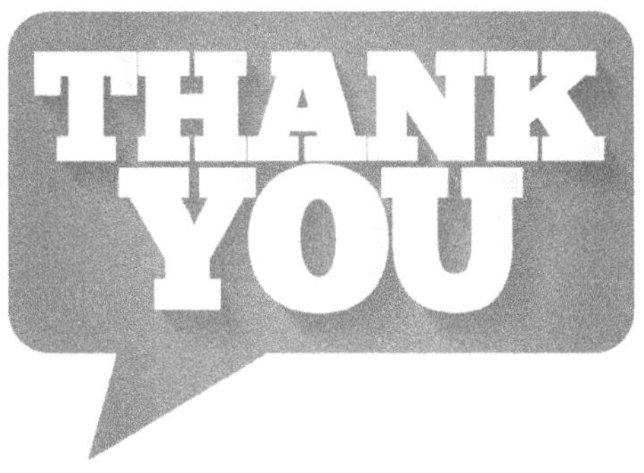

First and foremost, I would like to express my gratitude for downloading and reading my book. I hope that you found it informative and enjoyable. Writing books is my way of sharing my skills and expertise with readers like you.

I am aware that there are countless books available, and I am truly grateful that you chose mine. Your decision means a lot to me, and I am confident that you made the right choice.

If you could provide me with honest feedback about my book, it would make me even happier. Feedback is essential for growth and development. It helps me to improve the content of my book and generate new ideas for future publications. Who knows, your feedback might just spark an idea for my next book!

Thank you once again for taking the time to read my book, and I hope to hear from you soon.

Sincerely,

Martin Beasant